Contents

The One-Week Insomnia Cure

PROFESSOR JASON ELLIS

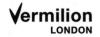

1 3 5 7 9 10 8 6 4 2

Vermilion, an imprint of Ebury Publishing,
20 Vauxhall Bridge Road,
London SW1V 2SA

Vermilion is part of the Penguin Random House group of companies
whose addresses can be found at global.penguinrandomhouse.com

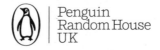

Copyright © Jason Ellis 2017

Jason Ellis has asserted his right to be identified as the author of this
Work in accordance with the Copyright, Designs and Patents Act 1988

First published in the United Kingdom by Vermilion in 2017

www.penguin.co.uk

A CIP catalogue record for this book is available from the British Library

ISBN 9781785040634

Printed and bound in Great Britain by Clays Ltd, St Ives PLC

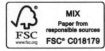

Penguin Random House is committed to a sustainable
future for our business, our readers and our planet.
This book is made from Forest Stewardship Council®
certified paper.

Acknowledgements

I have had some of the best mentors, formally and informally, in the world in terms of both the science, and practice, of Behavioural Sleep Medicine. In particular, I owe more than sincere thanks, even though I may not have said it at the time, and will always be immensely grateful to Simone de Lacy, Derk-Jan Dijk, Annette Sterr, Colin Espie, Michael Perlis, Donn Posner, Charles Morin and Dieter Riemann. Additionally, I have worked with some amazing colleagues in this field who have given me more to think about, and write about, than is humanly possible – Celyne Bastien (TSC), Michael Grandner, Sean Drummond, Anne Germain, Sara E, Cara Junquist, Kevin Morgan, Julia Newton, Vincent Deary, Wendy Troxel, Malcolm von Schantz, Rob Meadows, Bandana Saini, Janet Cheung, Renata Rhia, Alice Gregory, Jeanne Duffy and Nicola Barclay to name but a few. There are also the forgotten ones – i.e. previous students and trainees, who, as I have said many times in many locations, did all the work while I floated around the world talking about it. In particular, Greg Elder, Rachel Sharman, Zoe Gotts, Umair Akram, Samantha Man, Naomi Hynde, Charlotte Randall and Toby Cushing. I am delighted to say that many of you have, and whether you liked it or not, transcended the boundaries of mentor, colleague or trainee and become my friends. I must, must, must also thank my patients, both in research and clinic. You all own this book in one way or another. Either through your narratives, tweaking suggestions or critical but constructive feedback, I have learnt to be more as both a scientist and practitioner. I would also like to thank everyone at Penguin/Random House for the opportunity to write this book and, in particular, Sam Jackson, Katy Denny and Emma Owen for their support throughout the process and also

Jane Birch for keeping me editorially 'on point'. Believe it or not, I also have friends outside the sleep medicine arena and they are the ones who keep me 'grounded' and try, desperately, to keep me to a work–life balance, with very limited success. To that end, I will always be thankful for Harry (little man), Elissa, Luci and David, Brian and Icks, Chris W, Ari and the girls, Analiza and the boys, Maz, Phil and Georgie, Ren and Roseanne, Steve and Bill, Stevie, Kay and Bob, Tom and Lukas, Beth and Jeff, Beth and Hilary, Jean and Deb, Barbara and Terri, Sheila and Arthur, Lynne and Harry, Pam and Trevor, Andriy and Hanna, Alex and Rob and Blakey. To my families as well, both in the UK and the USA, thank you for being there even though I am lousy at calling! Also, to Jackie for keeping the house beautifully clean while I got on with that academicy 'stuff'. Together, the support of this enormous group of people is why you have this book and why I, I believe, have good mental health. Finally, to my significant other Dean, you are 'At Last' … nuff said!

The last acknowledgement I would like to make is to insomnia itself. Without you, as an unwelcome guest in my home, many years ago, I would not have started this journey …

Foreword

I will be upfront about one thing from the beginning, which, as you will see, I do a lot. The principles and techniques that this course is built upon are not mine. I have 'put together' the best combination, including some tweaked versions of my own, of what I believe, have seen and have used when working with people with insomnia to bring about the change we need. Along those lines, and where possible, I have acknowledged who, I believe, is the originator of that theory, method or technique (even when I have tweaked their technique mercilessly). I would also point out that, although I have mentioned an individual or group of individuals with respect to a particular theory, technique or method, that is not the sole contribution that individual has, or continues to make, to the study and practice of Behavioural Sleep Medicine. Through their research, teaching and practice, each of those individuals has moved the awareness, acceptance and refinement of courses, like this one, forward immensely. That being said, the structure of this course and the tweaks are mine and I have found that this approach, although others may feel free to disagree, is the best way to bring about the change that we need and to abolish insomnia in the short term and prevent it from happening again in the future. The last thing I would like to say at this point is this. Whilst I do understand that the title of this book could be considered controversial, and some might question the use of the term cure, it is my belief that we can manage an individual's insomnia symptoms, using the techniques that I will outline, in a week. Additionally, I believe we can prevent a sleep disturbance from developing into insomnia in the future. As such, it is in essence what we are doing through the management and prevention strategies outlined here.

How to Use This Book

Part 1

In Part 1 I will introduce you to some of the concepts that will help you understand what sleep is and how it works. The main purpose of Part 1 is that it will provide much of the groundwork for explaining why we will be doing the things that we do over the duration of the course. We will begin Part 1 by discussing the two main biological processes that affect when, where and how we sleep – the sleep homeostat (the biological drive to sleep) and the sleep/wake circadian rhythm (the internal body clock). I am then going to demonstrate how sleep disturbances and most sleep problems are caused by a mismatch between the sleep homeostat, the sleep/wake circadian rhythm and/or the environment we find ourselves in.

From there, we will look more closely at what insomnia is and how it develops and we will go through a series of questions to determine whether you have insomnia and, if so, if the course is appropriate for you. After that, I will introduce the concepts of sleep-related 'conditioned arousal' (the increasing levels of alertness and negative thoughts people with insomnia get when they get ready for bed or enter the bedroom) and 'cortical arousal' (your natural awakening threshold in the night) and show how both of these forms of arousal relate to sleep quality (how you feel in the morning based upon how you slept the previous night).

Although all of that may just sound like a really boring intellectual exercise, this first section of the book and, in particular, the information about insomnia (what it is, how it is defined and how it develops) are important to work through carefully. However, the discussion after that – Am I a Candidate for the Course? (page 61) – is probably the most important of all. Here, we will be going through an algorithm to determine what, if any, factors you may need to take into account before you can start the course or, indeed, if the course is right for you at all. You should not proceed with any part of the course until you have been through the algorithm and, if need be, made some necessary adjustments or sought additional support or help.

Following that, we will talk about pre-planning and sleep hygiene. The pre-planning stage and the sleep hygiene advice that I provide are not included in Part 2, which is the one-week course, but can definitely, if managed well, improve both the chances of success and level of improvement you will see on completion of the course. Finally, at the end of Part 1 I will introduce you to the Pre-course Sleep Diary, which you must complete before you start the course.

It is my intention that, by the time you are finished with Part 1, you will have a pretty good idea about whether or not you meet all the criteria for insomnia and whether the course is right for you, right now, and whether you should proceed to Part 2 or not. If you reach the end of Part 1, and it turns out that you do not have insomnia or that you are not a candidate for the course at this time, then it may be a good idea to talk to your General Practitioner (GP)/Primary Care Provider (PCP) or a Behavioural Sleep Medicine specialist (BSM) about your sleep. In the meantime, I would advise putting the sleep hygiene advice on page 86 into practice and completing a Pre-course Sleep Diary (see page 94). The diary will be really helpful for the GP/PCP or BSM to help determine what, if any, sleep problem(s) you may have and sleep hygiene is good for all of us, whether we have a sleep problem or not. Additionally, you may want to look at the information on Other Sleep Disorders (page 64), as this may give you an initial idea of what kind of sleep problem you may have.

SOME DEFINITIONS

SLEEP DISTURBANCE, SLEEP PROBLEM AND SLEEP DISORDER

You may notice that I use the terms 'sleep disturbance' and 'sleep problem' throughout. As this is deliberate, it is worth me explaining why I do this now. I define a sleep disturbance as having a period of poor sleep for a short amount of time, usually anywhere between three nights and two weeks. The reason I do this is because it is my belief that a brief disruption to an individual's sleep, especially in the case of a sleep disturbance caused by a stressor, is actually biologically adaptive and perfectly 'normal'. I will talk a lot more about that later. I use the term sleep problem when an individual's sleep has been poor for longer than two weeks but we don't know what the actual sleep problem is yet. Finally, later I will talk more about 'sleep disorders'. In these instances, not only has the poor sleep been around for more than two weeks, but we have identified the problem(s), based upon an assessment of the main symptoms that the individual has and, indeed, that individual's sleep.

INSOMNIAC OR PERSON WITH INSOMNIA?

I never use the term 'insomniac' but rather 'people with insomnia'. There is a good reason for this. I absolutely hate the term 'insomniac'. Although it may feel that insomnia is running your life, and that is a perfectly legitimate feeling, the term 'insomniac' suggests that the insomnia defines who you are and that, to my mind, is simply not the case. It is something you have that needs to be dealt with, not part of your identity. We would not call someone with chronic pain a 'painiac' so why the term 'insomniac' has been entered into our vocabulary I really do not understand.

Part 2

This comprises seven main components, which I will outline briefly below. The intention here is that, unless specified in Part 1 that you are not a suitable candidate for the course (for example, if you do not meet the criteria for insomnia) or that you need to make some alterations to the course, after going through the algorithm that I provide, you will work through a new section each day and apply the techniques from that section that same day/evening/night.

The Techniques

Day 1 – Sleep Rescheduling. We will use your Pre-course Sleep Diary to create your personal sleep schedule for the remainder of the course.

Day 2 – Stimulus Control. We will be looking to break the association between the bedtime routine, the bed and not being able to sleep.

Day 3 – Cognitive Control. We will examine ways of putting the day to bed before you go to bed to stop worry and frustration at night.

Day 4 – Cognitive Distraction Techniques. We will look at ways to stop your racing mind preventing you from being able to sleep at night.

Day 5 – Decatastrophising Sleep. We will look at techniques that help you identify and manage unrealistic and dysfunctional sleep-related thoughts.

Day 6 – Sleep Titration and Progressive Muscle Relaxation. We will look at how well all the previous techniques have worked for you in terms of your insomnia symptoms and start tailoring your sleep rescheduling schedule, if necessary. Additionally, we are going to look at the main relaxation technique that has been used with people with insomnia.

Day 7 – Maintaining Success and Relapse Prevention. Here we will look to the future and ways to manage your successes and protect yourself from having another episode of insomnia.

Cognitive Behavioural Therapy for Insomnia (CBT-I)

Together, these techniques make up the core of Cognitive Behavioural Therapy for Insomnia (CBT-I), or at least my version of it. So, where did these techniques come from and what is CBT-I?

CBT-I has been around for over 30 years and the research that it has been built upon is much, much older than that. In brief, CBT-I is the name for a collection of techniques that have all been shown, to varying degrees, to be helpful for people who have insomnia. All these techniques have been packaged together, in my view, for one main reason – because insomnia is not the same for every individual affected. As you will read later, insomnia can take many forms and be influenced or complicated by many different situations and personal circumstances. As such, adding all these techniques, at least the ones that we know make a difference for people with insomnia, together will help the broadest range of people who have insomnia.

There are two main aspects to CBT-I – cognitive and behavioural. The cognitive aspects are there to help us manage all the worries, concerns and anxieties that are related to our insomnia, in addition to helping us identify patterns in our thinking and coping which, although appearing logical and rational, may not actually be that helpful and, in some cases, may in fact be keeping the insomnia going. The behavioural aspect of CBT-I, on the other hand, looks at identifying and changing the habits, rituals and behaviours that we have developed, mainly in response to having insomnia, which may also be keeping the insomnia going.

Some people have got caught up in the 'What is more important – cognitive or behavioural?' debate but I tend to see these distinctions as rather artificial. If you are identifying and changing behaviours that are incompatible with sleep, you have to think about how best to do that and, if you are identifying and challenging negative thoughts and feelings about your sleep, it requires you to do something. What we do know is that, since the early studies on this combination of cognitive and behavioural techniques, more and more studies have been done (well over one hundred to date) and today CBT-I is a very well-defined, well-evidenced treatment for people with insomnia, whether they have insomnia alone or in combination with a variety of conditions and/or special circumstances. In fact, many organisations around the world related to health and healthcare suggest CBT-I should be the first option for treating people with insomnia and there is good reason for this.

Following the main part of the course (the CBT-I components) I have included Other Helpful Techniques (page 169). Here, we will look at a couple of other techniques – paradoxical intention and mindfulness for sleep and insomnia – that, although not part of a standard course of CBT-I, have been shown to be beneficial for people with insomnia over the years. These are not included to replace any section of the course but may be helpful additions that you can try at your leisure. By the end of Part 2 you will have learnt, and integrated into your life, each of the techniques that have been designed to help you get off to sleep quicker, stay asleep during the night and wake feeling more in control and refreshed.

Part 3

In Part 3 I will introduce a series of case studies of individuals with insomnia alongside another illness, disorder or condition. Throughout this section, where appropriate, I will highlight additional treatments and considerations that you may find helpful if you have another illness in addition to insomnia.

At the end of the book, I have included some tips on how to talk to your GP/PCP about sleep (see page 203) and how to locate a good BSM (see page 205).

The final thing that I would like to say at this point is, what you learn throughout this book is learnt for life. As you will see in Day 7 – Maintaining Success and Relapse Prevention (page 157), many, if not all, aspects of this course will be invaluable in managing your sleep, despite the challenges you face, from here on in.

What Can I Expect From This Book?

So, one question remains before we begin. What should I expect by the end of this book? I will be upfront with you about two things. The first is the likelihood that you will not be increasing how much time you sleep (your total sleep time) by very much by the end of this course. The second is that you are not likely to be sleeping as you did when you were a teenager either (unless you had problems during that time in which case you probably don't want to). So why bother?

In terms of total sleep time, we can all recall a night where we did not sleep that long but we still felt refreshed and alert in the morning. That is an issue of getting good-quality sleep, as opposed to sleep quantity, and that is the place we are aiming to get you to by the end of the book. Ask yourself this: would you prefer 6 hours of really good-quality sleep or 8 hours of really poor-quality sleep? I know which I would prefer.

And so, I am going to ask you to do the techniques outlined in Part 2 every day, in order to accomplish two things:

1. Increase your overall sleep quality
2. Reduce the amount of time that you are awake at night (the time it takes you to fall asleep and/or the amount of time you spend awake during the night or in the early hours of the morning).

If your only goal is to increase the amount of sleep you are getting, we will be addressing that too and all the techniques and strategies that you will be using will help accomplish that, but that change is likely to come after the course is finished. The point to remember is that we need to increase your sleep quality first and then it will take time to increase the quantity of sleep you can get and that is something that cannot be rushed. Otherwise you will end up with increased amounts of poor-quality sleep.

As for the second issue – sleeping like a teenager – that is simply never going to happen. I am sorry to tell you that but there are, as yet, no products, pills, courses or treatments available that will be able to take you back to that time in your life, at least in terms of your sleep. What you need to decide from this point and moving forward is what kind of sleeper you want to be in the future? That should be your goal.

PART 1

Sleep Basics

Sleep and Sleep Medicine

What Is Sleep?

We spend over a third of our lives doing it and when we do it 'normally' we tend to take it for granted. However, we soon realise its importance to our daily lives when we don't sleep well, even for just a couple of nights. So what is sleep? If you ever get the chance to watch someone sleeping, which although sounds a little creepy, I do quite a lot, you will probably conclude that there are three main outward physical signs of someone sleeping:

1. Closed eyes
2. Lying down
3. Being quiet (mostly).

These three signs, at first glance, would suggest sleep is quite a passive activity and for a long time this was believed to be the case. In fact it was not until the 1950s that it was first discovered that sleep was not just a single passive phenomenon but there were two main types of active sleep – Rapid Eye Movement sleep or REM sleep and non-REM sleep. Later studies showed that non-REM sleep was not just one single state, but could be characterised, by looking at the width (speed) and height (amplitude) of brainwave activity, into four 'distinct' stages: Stage 1 sleep–Stage 4 sleep. The reason I put the word distinct in quote marks is because, if you ever look at a sleep recording (a polysomnogram, which I will explain later – see page 43), the distinction between stages is not always as clear-cut as you would imagine, or would like, and involves some level of subjective interpretation, albeit by someone trained in analysing this kind of brainwave activity. However, from the point of discovery of the different stages of non-REM sleep onwards, scientists began to look beyond describing sleep to trying to understand how it works and why we, in addition to most if not all living things, do it.

Process C and Process S

In the 1980s Professor Alexander Borbély, a Swiss scientist, provided a framework to understand how sleep is regulated in humans. He suggested that sleep is a dynamic process that is largely regulated by the interaction between two internal mechanisms, the circadian rhythm and the sleep homeostat.

The circadian rhythm or, as it is also known, Process C, is, in essence, the body clock. The circadian rhythm produces roughly 24-hour cycles in many biological functions, including core body temperature, immune responsiveness, cortisol (stress hormone) secretion and digestion. For example, our core body temperature is, under most 'normal' circumstances, at its lowest (coldest point) in the early hours of the morning. Throughout the early morning and over the course of the day our temperature will gradually increase until the mid afternoon, where it will be at its highest (hottest point), before beginning to decrease again.

This pattern, although it may be altered in terms of the degree of change, tends to repeat irrespective of how much sleep we have had the night before. That said, whereas many other circadian rhythms such as core body temperature, cortisol secretion and immune response could be affected by certain events (for example, the temperature, cortisol and immune-response changes that are associated with an infection), the main hormone that regulates the sleep/wake circadian rhythm remains largely intact. That hormone is melatonin (the sleepiness hormone).

Put simply, melatonin is produced by the pineal gland in the brain and, as the amount produced increases, we become sleepier. During the day melatonin levels will be negligible, but they begin to rise in the latter part of the evening (usually about 2 hours before bedtime). This point is known as the 'sleep gate' or 'sleep onset zone' and melatonin production continues, with the highest concentrations being reached in the early hours of the morning, before they begin to decline again.

However, where we would naturally assume that the sleep/wake body clock in humans would be 24 hours, to correspond with our day, it is in fact slightly longer than that in most humans (around 24¼ hours) and there is quite a bit of variation between individuals. As such, where Process C is largely an internal (endogenous) mechanism, it is highly reliant on external (exogenous) cues to keep us regulated to 24 hours. From several years of research, three main factors that externally help regulate the sleep/wake circadian system have been identified, namely: light, food and exercise. For example, even small amounts of blue light at night can suppress the production of melatonin, making us more alert and potentially delaying our sleep onset (getting off to sleep). Here we get our first glimpse as to why there may be such a high prevalence of sleep disturbance in the general population. Reliance on these external factors that help regulate the sleep/wake circadian rhythm means that they can create a sleep disturbance, or at least worsen sleep if they are of insufficient magnitude (for example, limited access to natural light during the day) or exposure to these factors occurs at inappropriate times (for example, exercising just before bedtime). The good news is that if these three factors can disrupt the sleep/wake circadian rhythm, or Process C, then they can also be used, with some care, attention and pre-planning, to alleviate some sleep problems and this will be covered further in Sleep Hygiene (page 86), Other Sleep Disorders (page 64) and Day 7 – Maintaining Success and Relapse Prevention (page 157).

Process S

The other mechanism outlined by Professor Borbély is the sleep homeostat (Process S), which is our natural drive to sleep. When we wake the drive to sleep should be minimal. In other words, you should wake feeling alert and refreshed. As the day progresses our drive to sleep should build and build, reaching a peak in the evening (one of the reasons why we feel more tired as the day progresses). If the individual goes to bed during this peak time and sleeps through the night, the drive to sleep should be met and the process should start all over again the next morning. That said, if the drive to sleep is not met at this time, this drive (increasing levels of sleepiness) continues until we do eventually sleep. If this process of increasing sleepiness continues for some time, such as in the case of prolonged sleep deprivation (and by deprivation, in this instance, I mean not getting any sleep at all), sleep can sometimes occur involuntarily – known as a microsleep. When a microsleep occurs you involuntarily go into sleep, albeit for a brief amount of time, and your ability to attend to and react to your environment is reduced, which can be dangerous, especially if you are driving or doing something that requires a lot of attention or concentration at the time.

Perhaps more importantly to us, in the case of insomnia, is the scenario in which we have a limited amount of sleep drive built up (otherwise known as having insufficient sleep pressure) when it is time for us to go to bed. The main cause of insufficient sleep pressure at bedtime is napping in the daytime as the sleep drive is partially sated during the day and only begins to accumulate again from the point the nap is terminated.

The way I like to explain the impact daytime napping can have on night-time sleep is by using food as an analogy. The need to eat, like sleep, is regulated by an internal drive, in that the longer we go without food, the hungrier we get. In the case of food, we generally eat three times a day whereas we generally sleep only once, so we have to bear that in mind. Imagine a scenario in which we have an enormous breakfast at, say, 8am. Is this going to impact on our levels of hunger at lunchtime (noon)? Probably. We are not going to feel terribly hungry at lunchtime and we may end up skipping that meal. What about the impact of that big breakfast on dinner? It is not really going to affect our hunger levels at dinner, especially if we skipped lunch or just had a light snack. However, let's say that, instead, you had an enormous lunch (although I love buffets, they are the worst for overindulging at lunchtime, in my experience) at noon. Is that likely to impact on your hunger levels at dinnertime at, say, 7pm? Probably. You are not going to be as hungry as you would 'normally' be and you will be less likely to want, or be able, to eat a full meal.

What we have demonstrated here is how the amount of food we consume, at different times, can affect our ability to eat regular meals. If we translate that to sleep and say we have a long nap (a big meal) at lunchtime, are we going to be able to sleep (eat a full meal) as easily in the evening? Not really. But let's take this analogy one step further. What about a scenario in which you have a mid-morning snack? That is likely to impact on your hunger levels at lunchtime but not likely to impact on your hunger levels at dinnertime. But what if you had the snack at 6pm (an hour before dinner)? Is that going to impact on your hunger at dinnertime? Absolutely. The drive to eat has been sated before you even sit down to eat your meal. Translating that to sleep, even a small nap (snack) can have an impact on your drive to sleep at night but the level of interference this can have on your night-time sleep is largely dependent on how close you nap before bedtime. So, both long naps (big meals) and naps late in the day (evening snacking) reduce the drive to sleep at night and can make it more difficult to get off to sleep.

Environmental Factors

As I mentioned earlier, environmental factors can also play a part in the development of a sleep disturbance, sleep problem or sleep disorder by influencing either the sleep homeostat or the sleep/wake circadian rhythm. The most common environmental factor that I encounter in practice is people's work schedule, although any activity (including social activities) that results in either a reduced opportunity to sleep, beyond what you physically need, or sleeping outside your 'normal' bedtime (at night) could be considered an environmental factor.

We have to remember that environmental factors are not just restricted to those things that prevent us from going to bed when we physically need to; they also include any activity that results in us waking up earlier than we physically need to. This is one of the main challenges we face with a 24-hour society. With the increasing demands on our time, associated with the modern age, coupled with technological and industrial advances (particularly advances in lighting and communication), in many instances we are expected to be available almost all the time and sacrifice our sleep just to keep up with those demands. If we just look at cultural sayings such as 'you snooze you lose' or 'I will sleep when I am dead', they reinforce the viewpoint that sleep is a commodity that can be easily traded, in terms of quantity and timing, and by extension, quality. Even though we now know this is not the case and that the right amount of good-quality sleep can actually give us a competitive edge in so many ways, those terms and that basic sacrificing philosophy are still largely in evidence today.

Other environmental influences include things like people we share the bed with, traffic noise and streetlights at night. In fact, anything from our external world that can impact on us getting the amount of good-quality sleep we need, via the sleep homeostat or sleep/wake circadian rhythm, could be considered an environmental influence. As such, environmental factors can easily disrupt sleep by reducing our opportunity to get to sleep or remain asleep when our bodies want or need to.

Larks and Owls

It is worth talking about individual differences in the timing of the sleep/wake circadian rhythm at this point. Here, we are mainly talking about something called 'chronotypes'. You may have heard of people describing themselves as either morning types (larks) or evening types (owls), although the majority of us will sit somewhere in the middle (intermediate types). What chronotype refers to is an individual difference in the timing of the sleep/wake circadian rhythm that translates, behaviourally, to our preference and levels of productivity at different times of day. Morning types will prefer to get things done, especially more challenging things, earlier in the day whereas evening types will be more productive later in the day. Moreover, as we would expect, morning types will want to go to bed earlier whereas evening types will want to go to bed later. With respect to insomnia, being an evening type has been shown to increase the risk for developing insomnia, possibly because of the mismatch between our biological preference for going to bed late, and getting up late, and the responsibilities associated with our social world (such as having to get up earlier than we would like to go to school or work). The amount of mismatch that exists between our biological preference and the actual time that we go to bed or get up, due to the demands of our daily lives, is called our level of 'social jet lag'. That said, associations between eveningness and irregular sleep schedules, shorter sleep durations, less physical activity, increased alcohol and caffeine consumption and smoking have also been observed in evening types, which may also increase our vulnerability to developing insomnia. As such, it may be the influence of eveningness on behaviour, the high levels of social jet lag they experience or a combination of the two that make owls more vulnerable to developing insomnia than larks.

Couples

One of the other issues regarding chronotypes and insomnia, and the reason that I am talking about them here, is because of our significant others. If one of a couple is an extreme morning type and the other an extreme evening type, this mismatch in the couple's biological preference in the timing of going to bed and waking up can sometimes create a sleep disturbance, which, if not managed, can develop into a form of insomnia. I have seen this on more than one occasion, especially with newly formed couples when they decide to spend more than one or two nights a week together. Prior to that, in my experience, they 'live' with this disparity and go back to their 'normal sleep preference' on nights where they don't sleep together.

However, when they start sleeping together permanently, one partner will want to go to bed reasonably early (morning person), whereas the other partner will not be tired at that time (evening person). If they both go to bed at the same time (in this case, let's say earlier), as a lot of couples want to do, then it is going to be more difficult for the evening person to fall asleep and may result in that person developing a long-standing difficulty getting off to sleep.

What I do on these occasions is talk to the couple about creating a 'cuddle time'. I know it sounds a bit silly (I could not think of anything else to call it at the time), but it actually helps, not only with both partners' sleep but also, by extension, their relationship. In this case, the couple determines a bedtime, usually suited to the morning-oriented person, and the couple goes to bed for a specified amount of 'cuddle time' together. For the evening-oriented person, there should be no intention to sleep at that time, just to be there. As for how long 'cuddle time' should last, in my experience, between 15 and 20 minutes appears to work best.

The Interaction Between
Process C and Process S

The thing to remember here is that, while the sleep/wake circadian rhythm works largely independent of the amount of sleep you have had, the sleep drive continues accumulating until you have slept and only then will it be reset. So, all things being equal, during the day your body will be producing cortisol (and suppressing melatonin) to keep you awake and responsive and there should be little to no sleep drive to make you sleepy. During the evening the production of melatonin tends to coincide with a sufficiently high sleep drive to create what we call a 'sleep window' (a period of time when sleep is most likely to occur) with sleep very soon becoming the desired response. If you miss the window, which is usually the case when we deprive ourselves of sleep (the drive to sleep continues but you have stopped producing melatonin and started producing cortisol), then sleep will become less likely, and vice versa (if you are producing lots of melatonin but there is no drive to sleep, as in the case of napping late in the day).

In summary, dysregulation of either Process C or Process S (internally motivated by a change in physiology or externally motivated by the environment) has the capacity to create a sleep disturbance, which, if not corrected over time, can develop into a sleep problem. Additionally, as Process C and Process S work largely in concert throughout the 24-hour day, a significant mismatch between the two can also create a sleep problem (for example, the jet lag we associate with air travel occurs because of a rapid and significant mismatch being created between Process C and Process S and the environment).

Hence, one of the main questions asked of a patient by a Behavioural Sleep Medicine specialist is how they feel in the morning. Feeling refreshed is an indicator that the interaction between Process C and Process S is working fine, but if the individual reports feeling tired, sleepy and irritable, that is a sign that the individual is not getting sufficient amounts of good-quality sleep and it is usually something to do with Process C, Process S or the interaction, or lack thereof, between the two.

Normal Sleep

As I mentioned earlier, and contrary to early beliefs, sleep is a very active process. As we begin to get ready for sleep, overall brain activity does indeed slow down but it never fully stops, with different parts of the brain remaining active throughout the whole night while other parts of the brain become less (down regulating) or more (up regulating) active during the different stages of sleep.

How Does the Process of Sleep Work?

When we get into bed (if indeed you are sleeping in a bed, which I prefer), after a short amount of time, we should enter Stage 1 sleep. Stage 1 sleep is that warm cosy feeling you get when you are still largely awake, but you can feel your mind and body slowing down as you drift in and out of sleep. At this point, you are easily awoken and, if asked, you would probably say that you were awake.

As the night progresses (if you are sleeping at night which, of course, is also preferable) you will go from Stage 1 to Stage 2 sleep – a deeper form of sleep, at least when compared with being awake or in Stage 1 sleep. At the transition from Stage 1 to Stage 2 it is common to experience something called a 'hypnic jerk' or 'sleep start', which may, or may not, be accompanied by a visual hallucination. The hypnic jerk occurs because the muscles contract very quickly. It leaves you with a feeling of falling;

some people describe it as the sensation you get when you are climbing down the stairs and you don't realise there is one last step and stumble slightly or you step off a kerb too quickly. For most people, the hypnic jerk should only happen once, if at all, and is perfectly normal and natural, albeit a little bit disconcerting to you or potentially annoying to your significant other. If it happens more than once at sleep onset or if the jerk is sufficiently powerful to keep you awake then it is worth seeing a Behavioural Sleep Medicine specialist, as they may be able to help with that.

If all goes well in the transition from wake to sleep, you should then begin a consolidated period of Stage 2 sleep. Although considered a form of 'light sleep', Stage 2 sleep is characterised by slowing brain activity, compared with Stage 1, with occasional spikes, known as k-complexes, and bursts of rapid activity, known as sleep spindles. Although k-complexes and sleep spindles can be seen in the later stages of sleep – Stages 3 and 4 sleep – they begin during, and are used to define, the onset of Stage 2 sleep. Following Stage 2 sleep, you then progressively enter Stages 3 and 4 sleep, collectively known as Slow Wave Sleep (SWS), or deep sleep.

Our brain activity slows even further but the height (amplitude) of our brainwaves increases. It will be difficult to wake someone up from SWS and, if awoken, they will usually say that they were asleep. Again, all being well and following a consolidated period of SWS, you will then go back up into Stage 2 and Stage 1 sleep respectively. The reason we go from deep sleep back up to the lighter stages of sleep is thought to be a by-product of our evolution as a species. It is suggested that, even though we are physically asleep during these periods of light sleep, we routinely scan the environment for unusual noises just to make sure it is safe to continue sleeping. This makes sense, as it would be unwise to progress into a deep form of sleep, where we would be less responsive, if a sabre-toothed tiger or other predator entered our cave.

Following this period of light sleep you will begin your first consolidated period of Rapid Eye Movement (REM) sleep.

Interestingly, during REM sleep our brainwave patterns look very similar to those of being awake. During REM sleep, our heart rate will increase and blood pressure will rise, compared with the other stages of sleep, and we will also see short, shallow breathing, which can appear at first glance as laboured but is, in fact, quite normal. During this time the body should also be in a state of full paralysis and this is when the majority of our dreaming takes place.

This whole process, from Stage 1 sleep to REM sleep, takes 90–100 minutes (known as a full sleep cycle) and, once completed, the next cycle begins the process all over again, albeit with very small amounts of Stage 1 sleep. Whereas for the rest of the night (i.e. not including the first sleep cycle), Stage 1 and Stage 2 sleep don't tend to change much in terms of duration, during the first part of the night we maximise on large, consolidated periods of SWS and then, as the night progresses, the length of those periods of SWS becomes shorter and is replaced by longer, consolidated periods of REM sleep. So, you are most likely to wake from REM sleep, and consequently from a dream, than SWS in the morning. The diagram below shows how the different stages of sleep occur over a typical night.

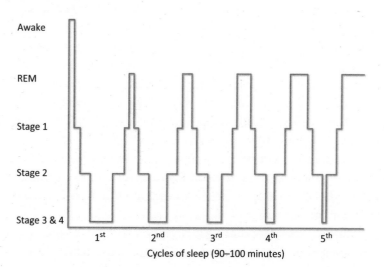

We know that getting the right amount of sleep is important for development, growth and repair and provides benefits in terms of overall mental and physical functioning, but what are the benefits in terms of each stage of sleep? Although we can examine each stage further to see the unique contribution each makes to our health and wellbeing, a great deal of the research in this area remains to be done, so we should be a little cautious about making too many generalisations at this point.

When it comes to Stage 1 sleep, we believe that it does not have a direct influence on health and wellbeing; rather, it is a period of time that gets our mind and body ready for the transitions that occur between sleep and wakefulness throughout the night and, as I mentioned, allows us to check the environment to make sure it is safe. This is probably why Stage 1 takes up a very small amount of our overall sleep time, at least in 'normal' sleepers (usually less than 5% of the total night).

In 'normal' sleepers, Stage 2 takes up approximately half the night and for a long time we did not really fully understand its true purpose. More recent research suggests that Stage 2 sleep, and in particular the k-complex and sleep spindle, may actually serve several very important functions: protecting deep sleep (by keeping the brain 'asleep' when there is a non-threatening external noise, for example), regulating sleep-related arousals (making sure the transitions from the end of one sleep cycle to the beginning of another don't wake us up), reviewing what has happened and what we have learnt today and preparing our memories for consolidation into long-term memory later on.

The Benefits of SWS

Together, SWS takes up between 13 and 23% of the overall night, although there are sex differences (younger women tend to have more SWS than younger men) and age-related changes (the amount of SWS we get declines from young adulthood to older adulthood) associated with the amount of SWS we get. So what does SWS do for us? Results from studies in which SWS has been manipulated (reduced or eliminated altogether) or under conditions in which SWS is naturally reduced, such as with some illnesses or medications, suggest that SWS protects, rejuvenates and revitalises our physical body. In particular we produce growth hormone during SWS, which is vital for growth and development in adolescents and helps repair damaged tissue and muscle, as we get older. Interestingly, SWS has more recently been associated with consolidating declarative memories. Declarative memories are those that we store and can recall, or 'declare' – for example, I know that x marks the spot. This makes sense, considering one of the purposes of Stage 2 sleep is to review what we have learnt today, getting it ready for long-term memory consolidation.

REM

REM accounts for approximately 20–25% of our sleep at night. REM has traditionally been associated with dreaming (although we now know that you can also be in non-REM sleep and still dream) and with consolidation of long-term procedural memory, the memory that knows how to do things – for example, I know how to build a fire. That said, new research has demonstrated an important additional benefit of REM – we clear out toxins from the brain during this time.

So it appears that nearly, if not all, the different stages of sleep are essential for a holistic balance between mind and body in terms of our sleep quality and its impact on our health and wellbeing.

You may notice that I use the word consolidated, here and throughout the book, a great deal when talking about sleep and health. The reason is that it is important to have consolidated periods of each sleep stage, especially SWS and REM sleep, to ensure you get good-quality sleep. Disruption of a sleep cycle means that the stage of sleep that you were in has been fragmented and it takes time to get back into that stage of sleep, if you can at all. In essence, there is a qualitative difference between 7 hours of uninterrupted sleep and the same amount of sleep that is fragmented, which will be reflected in how refreshed you feel in the morning. This is why I talk about improving sleep quality before we increase sleep quantity.

How Much Sleep Do I Need?

The media tend to report that the average adult needs approximately 8 hours of sleep a night, although you may have come across other figures that have been bandied about, such as 7 hours or 7½ hours. Before we get worried or upset that we are not sleeping exactly 8 hours, every night, the first thing to remember is that these figures are all based upon averages. Think about it this way: the average shoe size in the United States of America for men is 10½ and for women 9. If we produced only shoes that were either 10½ or 9, then we would have a lot of people walking around barefoot!

Here, we have to consider individual differences in the amount of sleep we need. Some of us will need more sleep and others of us will need less. As for the specific 8-hour issue, there are guidelines, published in 2015 by the National Sleep Foundation (NSF), on the optimal range of sleep need, by age category, which I have adapted and provided below. As you will see, there is no definitive number of hours needed at any point over the lifespan. What the NSF outlines are 'recommended', 'potentially appropriate' and 'not recommended' ranges, just like we have ranges for our calculations for body mass index. In line with the NSF, I generally talk about a range for sleep need anywhere between 6 hours and 11 hours for younger adults (between 18 and 25 years old), 6 hours and 10 hours for adults (between 26 and 64 years old) and between 5 hours and 9 hours for older adults (65 years old and older). Anyone reporting an amount of sleep outside those ranges tends to signal a red flag to me to further investigate, and not necessarily for insomnia.

Recommended (fully shaded) and Maybe Recommended (partially shaded) Hours Sleep

AGE	NOT RECOMMENDED
NEW BORN 0–3 months	Less than 11 hours / More than 19 hours
INFANT 4–11 months	Less than 10 hours / More than 18 hours
TODDLER 1–2 years	Less than 9 hours / More than 16 hours
PRE-SCHOOL 3–5 years	Less than 8 hours / More than 14 hours
SCHOOL AGE 6–13 years	Less than 7 hours / More than 12 hours
TEENAGER 14–17 years	Less than 7 hours / More than 11 hours
YOUNG ADULT 18–25 years	Less than 6 hours / More than 11 hours
ADULT 26–64 years	Less than 6 hours / More than 10 hours
OLDER ADULT 65+ years	Less than 5 hours / More than 9 hours

So, is it important to find out how much sleep you need as an individual? Absolutely, as either too little or too much sleep, over a long term, can be detrimental to our health and wellbeing. The acid test to determine whether you are getting the sleep you need is to ask yourself how you feel in the morning, between 20 and 40 minutes after waking. If you feel tired, sleepy or unrefreshed, then there is likely to be a problem with the quality, quantity or timing of your sleep that needs further investigation.

Determining How Much Sleep You Need

While our sense of being unrefreshed in the morning tells us that we are not getting either the right amount of good-quality sleep or that our sleep timing is off, it does not really help with finding out how much sleep we actually need. There is one way in which you can try to determine how much sleep you need, yourself, without lots of equipment or a specialist, but I would NOT recommend trying this while doing the course, perhaps later when you are sorted and sleeping better. The best way to do this, that I know of, is to take a week out of life (not an easy thing to do at the best of times). Put another way, there should be no distractions that would force you to go to bed or get up at a certain time (for example, children, work commitments, partners, pets, alarm clocks).

For that week, listen to your body and go to bed and get up at whatever time you want each day. In other words, go to bed when you are sleepy and get up when you naturally awaken. During that week you should also record how long you slept for each night. The key is to look at the last three nights that you record. Those three nights should be averaged and that will give you a good indication of how much sleep you, as an individual, need at this point in time. For example, if I slept 7½ hours on Night 5, 7 hours on Night 6 and 7¼ hours on Night 7, my average sleep need would be 7¼ hours.

Why the last three nights? For the first four nights of your 'experiment' you will be acclimating to this new routine and, at the same time, getting rid of any pre-existing sleep debt or social jet lag. So, the first four nights are not going to be representative of your actual sleep need, whereas the last three are going to be a more accurate assessment. Remember that number will only be indicative of how much sleep you need at this point in your life.

This leads me to a brief discussion on age-related changes in sleep need. As we saw from the recommendations from the NSF earlier, there are some meaningful changes in the amount of sleep we need over the lifespan. But why is this? Newborn babies, toddlers, children and adolescents need more sleep than adults, and certainly more SWS and REM sleep, to help them grow and develop both physically and mentally. What we do see, however, is that sleep needs don't really tend to change much when we reach, and progress through, adulthood.

That said, there are several factors that can make sleep quantity, quality and sleep timing more of an issue for older adults. Primarily, the efficiency of both the sleep/wake circadian rhythm and sleep homeostat can decline in older adulthood and, as a result, we produce less melatonin and have fewer periods of consolidated sleep (more sleep fragmentation). Additionally, the amount of each sleep stage (sleep architecture) changes with normal ageing, with older adults spending more time in the lighter stages of sleep, as opposed to SWS or REM sleep. Older adults will also tend to go to bed earlier, wake early in the morning and nap during the day, although the reasons for this are less well understood and it may be a combination of physical changes in sleep mechanisms, that I just mentioned, and changes in environmental circumstances (for example, retirement). We do know that, as we progress through early adulthood, a lot of older adults become more morning orientated (lark-like). In essence, it appears, at least at first glance, that older adults need roughly the same amount of sleep as younger adults, but are more vulnerable to developing sleep problems, such as insomnia, due to many of these normal changes in their sleep physiology. One of the other main issues for older adults is increased levels of illness and medication, which can impact on how much sleep they obtain and the quality of the sleep they are getting.

What Are the Consequences of Too Little or Too Much Sleep?

I have mentioned sleep debt, which we all have to some degree. When we refer to sleep debt we are talking about how far we are between how much sleep we need and how much we are getting, irrespective of the cause. The difficulty here is that, although a sleep debt can be paid back, with some careful consideration over time, many of us just keep accumulating a sleep debt and have forgotten what good sleep is like. Alternatively, we try to repay all our weekday sleep debt at the weekend, which can disrupt the relationship between the sleep homeostat and the sleep/wake circadian rhythm by the time we reach Monday. But is a sleep debt a problem? Certainly, the consequences of getting too little sleep has been a hot topic in the media recently, with research suggesting that those who don't get enough sleep tend, in the long run, to become ill. Relationships between shorter sleep durations and illnesses including diabetes, heart disease, hypertension, depression, obesity and certain cancers have all been observed.

So, what about sleeping too much, can that be just as harmful? The answer, although less well studied than too little sleep, appears to be yes. Associations between longer sleep durations and illnesses, similar to many of those associated with shorter sleep durations (for example, diabetes, heart disease, depression, obesity and back pain) have all been observed. Why does this happen? There are two proposed pathways by which either too much or too little sleep is believed to affect your health – a direct pathway and an indirect pathway.

In the direct pathway hormones that regulate your stress response (cortisol), feelings of hunger and feeling full (ghrelin and leptin) and your ability to repair and respond to illness (innate immune response) become dysregulated when you have slept more or less than you need. In the long term these imbalances, and our bodies' attempts to correct them, will make us more susceptible to becoming ill. Certainly, we know that sleep deprivation tends to make us crave high-fat, sugar and carbohydrate snacks, especially in the afternoons. The indirect pathway suggests that too much or too little sleep impacts on our mood and decision-making ability, making us more likely to make unhealthy choices (increased sedentary behaviour, increased alcohol consumption, increased food consumption) which in the long term can lead to illnesses and diseases.

That said, it is important to remember that many of these studies have been unable to determine whether it is the illness that is influencing the length of our sleep or whether it is sleeping longer, or shorter, than is necessary is affecting our health. The key point for you to remember here, especially when hearing the reports in the media about the research that shows all the damage that too little or too much sleep causes, is that in many cases they are talking about research which has used sleep deprivation (experimentally keeping people awake) or sleep extension (experimentally keeping people in bed) to demonstrate these links. Sleep deprivation and sleep expansion are not the same things as insomnia. Yes, the concepts are related in that sleep deprivation and insomnia are focused on less amount of sleep than we consider 'typical' or 'normal', but, when we are talking about sleep deprivation, that usually means either no sleep at all or, when we are talking about partial sleep deprivation, we are usually talking about a person's sleep being restricted to 4 hours a night or fewer. It is unusual for someone with insomnia to sleep fewer than 4 hours a night and certainly not regularly over a long period of time. All that said, there have now been quite a few studies that demonstrate, over the long term, that having insomnia is not good for our physical or psychological health, with the most amount of evidence suggesting that having insomnia increases the risk of developing depression in the future. However, as with the studies on sleep deprivation, we have to be mindful that there are many other complicating factors, such as illnesses, alcohol use, sleep-medication use and a prior history of shift work, as a few examples, that may be independently contributing to this relationship.

What Are the Benefits of Good Sleep?

Whereas it is quite easy to get fixated on the negative aspects of a sleep debt, poor sleep and insomnia, which we can sometimes do, I always prefer to talk about the benefits of good sleep instead. What I mean by good sleep is when the quality, quantity and timing of the sleep you are getting matches your biological sleep need. We know that people who sleep well tend to be physically healthier overall and more able to fight infection, combat stress and control their blood pressure. Additionally, sleeping well has been shown to be associated with improved dieting performance both in terms of reduced body fat (poorer sleepers tend to lose muscle mass first) and a reduced number of 'slips' while dieting. Interestingly, these physical benefits are not just limited to the self, as research has shown that when people have slept well, others perceive them as more healthy, younger and more attractive. I suppose that is the reason it is called 'beauty sleep'. However, the benefits of good sleep go way beyond protecting or accentuating our physical health and I have compiled a list that demonstrates some of the additional benefits, that we know of, in terms of good sleep health:

- Increased ability to learn and remember information
- Increased ability to concentrate

- Increased creativity
- Increased ability to evaluate, and respond to, risk
- Increased belief in our ability to accomplish goals (self-efficacy)
- Increased energy and stamina
- Increased sexual drive
- Increased satisfaction with relationships
- Improved physical performance
- Improved mood.

As we can see, good sleep can confer benefits to all areas of our lives (social, emotional, psychological and physical). Even in people who would classify themselves as 'normal' or 'typical' sleepers there is always the possibility of improvement, for them to become good sleepers. In these instances, good sleep hygiene (see page 86), knowing what our sleep needs are (see page 25) and keeping to a regular sleep/wake schedule (going to bed and getting out of bed at similar times throughout the week) are the main keys to getting from 'normal' sleeper to good sleeper.

What Is Insomnia?

In its broadest sense insomnia is usually described as a problem of not getting enough sleep. That said, the picture is a little more complex than that, as a problem of not getting enough sleep can happen for a multitude of reasons, many unrelated to what we actually define as 'insomnia'. On the flip side, there are many diseases, disorders and conditions where poor sleep is present but individuals tend to think of the poor sleep as part of the illness as opposed to insomnia in its own right. As we know, insomnia can co-exist with any number of illnesses and conditions and in many cases when you manage, control or cure the illness (medically or otherwise) the insomnia can remain.

What Do We Classify as Insomnia?

When we classify any illness or disorder, including insomnia, we tend to use a diagnostic algorithm, like a checklist, that allows us to identify someone with the illness while, at the same time, ruling out other, albeit similar, illnesses. That way we can give the right treatment to the right patient, saving time and money. In the case of insomnia we have three sets of diagnostic algorithms to use – *The International Classification of Diseases*, by the World Health Organization; *The Diagnostic and Statistical Manual of Mental Disorders*, by the American Psychiatric Association (*DSM*, 5th edition); and *The International Classification of Sleep Disorders* (*ICSD*, 3rd edition), by the American Academy of Sleep Medicine. Thankfully, today all three tools use pretty much the same criteria to inform their algorithms, outlined below, although it has not always been the case:

1. A complaint, by the individual, of a difficulty in getting off to sleep, a difficulty in staying asleep or a difficulty of waking earlier than required in the morning without the ability to go back to sleep
2. The difficulty should exist despite adequate opportunity to sleep
3. The difficulty should be present for at least three nights per week
4. The difficulty should be present for at least three months
5. The difficulty should result in distress and/or disruption to daily functioning
6. The difficulty should not be adequately explained by another illness, disease, substance or better explained by another sleep disorder.

The first questions I tend to get when I outline these criteria to my students or trainees, when teaching about diagnosing insomnia, are 'Does the individual have to meet all six criteria to have insomnia?' and 'Is the order of the criteria important?' The answer to both questions is generally yes, with a couple of caveats, which I will outline in more detail when we go through each criterion. What I will say, is the reason we have the criteria dictated in this way is because we need to create the optimal balance between the sensitivity (making sure that people with the condition – in this case insomnia – are diagnosed correctly) and specificity (making sure that people who do not have the condition – in this case insomnia – are not misdiagnosed as having insomnia) of the algorithm.

So, the first criterion has very high sensitivity, but has low specificity. In other words, while most, if not all, people with insomnia will have a complaint with their sleep that is a problem of getting off to sleep, staying asleep or waking too early in the morning, many of the individuals with those complaints will have a problem with their sleep that is not insomnia. Conversely, all the other criteria, especially when combined, have high specificity to differentiate someone with insomnia from someone with a different kind of sleep problem. So, as you can see, the ordering is important, at least in terms of the first criterion, as it acts like a funnel, taking in the broadest number of people with sleep problems using the first criterion and then filtering down, using all the other criteria, to determine who does and who does not have insomnia.

Let's look at each criterion individually:

The First Criterion

The first criterion, otherwise known as the principal complaint, makes perfect sense; the individual has to report a problem, as they would with most illnesses or conditions. However, what this first point also does is tell us that there are potentially three (or more if you include a mixture of two or all three problems) different types of insomnia – problems getting off to sleep (known as initial insomnia), problems staying asleep (known as middle insomnia) and waking too early in the morning (known as late insomnia).

Is this important for you to know what type of insomnia you have for the course? Not really as the course works for all these types of insomnia, but it is helpful to know which you have so you can see how the course is impacting on your main problem(s). The question that tends to come up a lot when I outline the first criterion to individuals with insomnia is 'How much of a problem should there be for it to be classified as "insomnia"?' That is a tricky one, as none of the diagnostic algorithms covers this and they largely rely on the individual to determine whether, for them, their sleep is sufficiently problematic to seek help. That said, there are some general guidelines about how much of a problem there has to be to be classified as insomnia but we have to be mindful that these have been used mainly for research purposes.

For example, there is the 30/30 rule (if it takes you more than 30 minutes to get off to sleep or you are awake for more than 30 minutes during the night or in the morning) then, if all other conditions are met, it is likely to be insomnia. Personally, at least in terms of treatment, I believe that if you feel your sleep is a problem then it is a problem worth investigating, irrespective of how much time it takes you to get off to sleep or how long you are awake during the night.

The Second Criterion

This is an interesting one and is generally used to differentiate those with voluntary sleep problems (where the course is NOT indicated) from those with insomnia (where the course IS indicated). In essence, if you don't leave yourself enough time to sleep then the likelihood is that you are going to have a problem with your sleep. That does not necessarily make it insomnia but rather an environmentally determined problem of short sleep (otherwise known as Insufficient Sleep Syndrome).

It is not surprising that we are seeing more and more of this kind of sleep problem as we tend to sacrifice sleep more and more to keep up with the demands of a 24-hour society, as I mentioned earlier. The question to ask yourself here, to differentiate insomnia from Insufficient Sleep Syndrome, is how you sleep on days that you don't have commitments (for example, on non-work days or on holiday)? If you, more often than not, sleep well on those nights, the problem is more likely to be a case of not getting enough sleep as opposed to insomnia per se.

There may be one other situation that, albeit a little tricky to identify, could be causing your sleep problem through a lack of getting enough time to sleep. The reason I say this is a little trickier is that you may not explicitly be aware of it. I have never encountered this with someone who reports initial insomnia, as I am pretty sure they would be aware of it, but I have come across this with a few individuals who report middle or late insomnia. This is when something in the environment regularly creates an awakening but the individual is not altogether aware of what has woken them up. It may be the central heating coming on, a neighbour noisily arriving home from a night shift or slamming the front door when going to work for an early shift, or even an early train or aeroplane.

How do you identify this specific type of Insufficient Sleep Syndrome (I don't classify it as insomnia as it, to me, is a different kind of sleep problem)? The first clue I get is when I ask about the timing of the awakening(s). If an individual, with what appears to be either middle or late insomnia, reports that they wake up at approximately the same time every night, this suggests to me, at least as one possibility that needs investigating further, that there may be something in the environment that is causing them to wake up at that time. What I do in that instance is ask the individual to conduct an experiment of his or her own. Set your alarm five minutes before this exact time of awakening, just for a night or two, and see what happens. If there is something in the environment that is creating this problem then being awake at that time will help you identify what it is and then it can be addressed. Alternatively, if you don't fancy being awake you can set your phone, or another recording device, to start recording at that exact time and you can then review it at your leisure for any unusual noises.

The Third Criterion

The third criterion takes into account night-to-night variability in sleep. Although this has only been the subject of investigation, in insomnia, since the early 2000s, we now know that both 'normal' sleepers and individuals with insomnia have a night-to-night pattern in their sleep whereby even the most hardened person with insomnia will have a reasonable night's sleep once in a while and a 'normal' sleeper will have a poor night of sleep once in a while. This cut-off point of three nights per week allows us to differentiate between these two groups, but it also underscores the need for monitoring our sleep over successive days and weeks so that we can get a more accurate picture of what the problem with your sleep is (see Pre-course Sleep Diary and On-course Sleep Diary, pages 94 and 119).

The Fourth Criterion

This is probably the most debated criterion of all and is presumably used to differentiate acute insomnia (fewer than three months) from chronic insomnia (three months or more). Previous versions of the diagnostic algorithms have suggested a duration criterion ranging from one month to six months and no strong rationale has ever been provided for the current criterion of three months. The good news is that there is research currently underway in the United States of America (Dr Michael Perlis) and in the United Kingdom (myself) that will hopefully provide the answer of when a sleep disturbance becomes a sleep disorder (in this case insomnia) but the bad news is, as yet, we do not know.

Does it matter? As a scientist, I would say yes, but as a practitioner, not really. What I would say is that if you have had insomnia for two weeks, or fewer, then the course is NOT suitable at this time. I have two reasons for saying this:

1. The course has never been tested with people who have had this kind of sleep disturbance for such a short amount of time and so we don't know if it would do more harm than good
2. In my view, a sleep disturbance lasting less than two weeks is probably a normal biological reaction to stress as opposed to insomnia per se.

If someone who had insomnia for two months (still during the acute phase) wanted to see me for treatment, would I see them? Absolutely. In my view, the main rationale for a duration criterion would be so that we could devise shorter, quicker treatment strategies that would prevent the development of chronic insomnia. This is something we (my colleagues and I in the UK, and Dr Anne Germain) have been working on that I am going to share with you later (see Managing a Sleep Disturbance on page 166 and Managing Acute Insomnia on page 167).

The Fifth Criterion

The fifth criterion is really helpful in allowing us to differentiate between people with insomnia and those who may biologically need less sleep to function (biological short sleepers). As you saw earlier, we are all different and some of us need more sleep, or indeed less sleep, than others. If it is the case that you are a biological short sleeper, as opposed to having insomnia, then you should not have a significant daytime complaint. In other words, the amount of sleep you are getting should not really be causing you much distress or interfering with your day-to-day activities. A problem for short sleepers arises because in many cases these individuals do not know that they are biological short sleepers and they spend too much time in bed, most of it awake. How do you know if you are a biological short sleeper? It's a good question. Again, there is not a great deal of research in this area, with some notable exceptions in the work of Dr Julio Fernandez-Mendoza and Dr Michael Grandner, but from the research that does exist, the generally agreed definition includes regularly sleeping fewer than 6 hours without significant daytime distress or complaint. I would add to that and say sleeping anywhere between 5 and 6 hours regularly, without significant complaint.

The Sixth Criterion

The final criterion deserves some explanation. In the past, when someone with insomnia presented herself or himself with any other illness, condition or disorder (be it physical, psychological, medication- or substance-related, or another sleep disorder), the insomnia was automatically seen as a 'secondary' symptom to the underlying other condition, the thought being that, if the underlying other condition was managed appropriately, then the insomnia would just go away on its own.

That distinction no longer applies as we now know that in the majority of cases of insomnia co-occurring with another condition, successful management of the other condition does not necessarily resolve the insomnia and the insomnia needs to be assessed and treated in its own right. The way I interpret and approach this criterion is with one main question with one follow-up question. Did the insomnia start around the same time as the other condition or illness manifested? And, if so, is the other condition or illness now being successfully managed? If the answer to the first question is no or the answer to both questions is yes then we can go ahead with the full assessment for the course (see Am I a Candidate for the Course?, page 61). If the answer to the first question is yes but the answer to the second question is no, then it is possible that the other illness may adequately explain the insomnia, so I would recommend seeking treatment for the other illness or condition, from your

GP/PCP, before starting the course, just to make sure the other illness or condition is not adequately explaining the insomnia.

Under this algorithmic definition of insomnia we estimate that about 10–15% of the general population will have chronic insomnia (insomnia that has lasted over three months) at any given point in time and over a third of us (36%, according to research that my colleagues and I have undertaken) will have an episode of acute insomnia (between two weeks and three months) in any given year. The important thing to remember here is you are not alone. It may feel that way, as insomnia tends to be a very isolating experience and one that people don't tend to talk about (we talk about sleep a lot but we don't talk a great deal about sleep disorders and insomnia, in particular).

Insomnia Subtypes

As I mentioned earlier, there are the three types of insomnia (initial, middle and late), but it does not end there. We also talk about three main subtypes of insomnia:

1. Idiopathic Insomnia
2. Psychophysiologic Insomnia
3. Paradoxical Insomnia.

Although subtypes are not generally included in a routine assessment for insomnia, as one of them is particularly relevant to whether CBT-I, and indeed this course, is right for you, I always assess for subtypes in my research and practice and have included them here.

Idiopathic Insomnia, as the name suggests, is a form of lifelong insomnia. The individual has had insomnia since child-hood with few, if any, periods of brief remission.

Psychophysiologic Insomnia is a subtype of insomnia that is usually triggered by a specific stressful event or series of annoy-ing or irritating circumstances and is generally accompanied by evidence of conditioned arousal to the bedroom and/or pre-sleep routine, or even just the thought of bedtime, accompanied by a general preoccupation with sleep throughout the day. What do we mean by conditioned arousal? I will discuss this in detail later (see page 55), but for now we will say that it is the negative thoughts, feelings and emotions that someone with Psychophysiologic Insomnia automatically has when they are asked to think about or discuss their sleep or, indeed, when they go to bed.

Paradoxical Insomnia is an interesting subtype of insomnia and, albeit more rare than the other two, deserves some special attention. Paradoxical Insomnia occurs when there is a significant mismatch between what the individual perceives their sleep to be like and what it physically looks like. Now the first thing to say about this is that individuals with Paradoxical Insomnia are not crazy and they are not telling lies. Although we don't fully understand Paradoxical Insomnia, we know it is a real phenomenon and we believe, although there is limited research being done on the topic, that these individuals have a capacity for heightened sensory processing during sleep. In other words, they may appear to be physiologically asleep but parts of the brain are more active than we would expect and the individual is still attending to the environment, albeit to a reduced extent (see Cortical Arousal on page 58 for a detailed explanation). As such, people with Paradoxical Insomnia perceive themselves as awake when it would appear, by objectively measuring their sleep, that they are in fact asleep.

How do you know whether you have Paradoxical Insomnia? It is a tough question, as we still don't fully understand it and there are no accepted rules on how much of a mismatch has to be there for a diagnosis, as we all have a mismatch to some degree, so I use two rather conservative rules, just to be on the safe side:

1. If an individual reports involuntarily not sleeping at all on any given night in a week
2. If an individual reports involuntarily sleeping four hours, or fewer, on three or more nights per week.

In cases where either of these are reported I would suggest looking to confirming the presence, or absence, of Paradoxical Insomnia through a Behavioural Sleep Medicine specialist. They will be able to arrange a test, or series of tests, to determine whether and how much of a mismatch exists, using an objective sleep assessment device (actigraphy or polysomnography), or whether there is some other issue that may need special consideration before you can complete the course, if appropriate.

For each subtype, the individual will still need to meet all six criteria for insomnia but the course will vary depending upon which subtype of insomnia you have. While the full course is suitable for individuals with Idiopathic Insomnia or Psychophysiologic Insomnia, subject to the algorithm assessment on page 62, it is not the case for people with Paradoxical Insomnia who will do a modified version of the course (see page 103).

As I have just mentioned them, now would be a good time to talk about actigraphy and polysomnography and their relevance to insomnia, as both are particularly relevant for Paradoxical Insomnia, and will be mentioned again in Part 3. Both techniques allow us to objectively measure sleep with differing degrees of sophistication.

Actigraphy

Actigraphy uses an actigraph to measure sleep. The actigraph is a device, usually worn on the wrist, and looks a lot like a watch. Actigraphy uses a specific form of accelerometer designed to detect movement, through two or sometimes three polarised magnets, and translates that information, using a series of algorithms, into data about whether an individual is asleep or awake. In its simplest form, stillness equates to being asleep whereas movement implies wakefulness. In addition to basic information about that night's sleep, such as how long it took the individual to get off to sleep, how many times and for how long they were awake during the night, and for how long the individual actually slept comparative to how much time they spent in bed, the data that can be gathered from actigraphy, over time, can also tell us about an individual's sleep/wake pattern which can provide a crude marker of the stability and, to a lesser degree, the phase of the individual's sleep/wake circadian rhythm.

Polysomnography

What basic actigraphy cannot tell us is about the quality of an individual's sleep or how much time the individual spent in each of the different stages of sleep (the individual's sleep architecture). That is where polysomnography (PSG) comes in.

Full PSG is far more complex than actigraphy and involves several electrodes placed on the scalp, two behind the ears and sometimes one, two or even three across the forehead (Electroencephalography). There will also be one electrode placed a little above the right eye and another a little below the right eye (Electrooculography), two on the chest (Electrocardiography), one on the chin, two on the jaw and two on each leg, between the ankle and knee (Electromyography). Additionally, there will usually be two chest belts, a nasal transducer and a nasal cannula, which measure how well you are breathing, and a pulse oximeter on the finger to measure oxygen levels in your blood (blood oxygen saturation levels).

That is a lot of sensors, but how does it all work? The Electroencephalography (EEG) measures brainwave activity by enhancing, using a paste that conducts, and then recording the speed (frequency) and height (amplitude) of electrical signals in different parts of the brain. In order to do this effectively, the electrodes behind the ears act as reference points. If you feel behind your ear, just above the lobe (the mastoid), you will notice it is quite bony. As electrical signals cannot penetrate through this bone, we can measure the strength of the electrical signals from the scalp in relation to a place where there should be no signals and this allows us to correct for any false signals created by movements or other things that can interfere with the recording (such as background noise).

The electrooculography (EOG), together with the chin and jaw electrodes (electromyography), measure levels of muscle tension (tone) and allows us to differentiate wakefulness from REM sleep which, as I said earlier, can look very similar in terms of brain-wave activity alone. What we should be seeing in REM sleep is no muscle tone from the chin and jaw. The electromyography (EMG) on the legs also measures muscle tone and allows us to detect unusual leg movements or twitches during the night and the electrocardiography lets us monitor the electrical activity of the heart in a similar way to the EEG, which, in addition to iden-tifying abnormalities in the heart (heart rate or rhythm), can also give us an indication of whether the individual is asleep or awake.

All these signals, including the measures of breathing (res-piratory effort and flow) and blood oxygenation, are then digitised into waveforms and scored by someone trained in polysomnography. As each stage of sleep is characterised by changes in brainwave activity (frequency and amplitude), muscle tone (muscle tone reduces when we go to sleep, progressively reducing through deep sleep, and should be non-existent in REM sleep), heart activity and breathing, we can then identify how much of each stage of sleep someone has had, including how much consolidation of each sleep stage has occurred throughout the night, and any abnormalities or events that may be disrupting sleep.

In the case of a suspected case of Paradoxical Insomnia, the likelihood is that actigraphy will be used unless it is unavaila-ble or another sleep disorder or physical condition is suspected to sit alongside the Paradoxical Insomnia. In those cases PSG is likely to be used. Outside detecting cases of Paradoxical Insomnia, both actigraphy and PSG are not generally used with people with insomnia unless something else is suspected and in those cases the PSG or actigraphy will be used to rule out other sleep disorders or conditions that may look like insomnia. There are several reasons why we don't tend to use PSG, and to a lesser extent, actigraphy when we are dealing with individuals with Idiopathic or Psychophysiologic insomnia.

Primarily, and as you will have seen from the diagnostic criteria on page 33, insomnia is largely a self-reported problem. Because there are such individual differences in sleep need, in addition to the sex and age differences in how much sleep we need, it is quite difficult to determine how much of a sleep problem there would have to be for it to be diagnosed as insomnia. Add to the fact that, as I said earlier, insomnia is not the same for everyone, it would be difficult to suggest what would have to be outside the normal range in the PSG for it to be a case of insomnia. Moreover, lots of other things can influence what information we can get from a PSG, including medication use, drug use and alcohol use in addition to levels of social jet lag and sleep debt; as such the picture is not going to be all that clear.

Finally, access to PSG is quite limited and it is quite an expensive procedure. As we, as is always the case in a diagnosis of insomnia, have to record sleep over a period of time – remember the diagnosis for insomnia requires for it to be present for at least three nights per week – the costs and logistics associated will measuring sleep, via PSG, would be immense. All that said, there is some fantastic work being undertaken by Professor Dieter Riemann and his team, that is trying to determine whether we can detect PSG abnormalities that characterise insomnia, so watch this space.

How Insomnia Develops

We have seen how insomnia is diagnosed and had an introduction to the various types and subtypes of insomnia, but how does insomnia start and why does it go from a few poor nights of sleep (sleep disturbance) to a condition that feels relentless and permanent (insomnia as a sleep disorder)?

A scientist named Professor Art Spielman introduced the most comprehensive model of the development of insomnia in 1987. Although he modified his model later on, we are going to stick with the original, as it is, in my view, visually a much better way for you to identify how insomnia could have developed, and is being maintained, using your own personal circumstances and experiences.

One question you may ask is why are we going to talk about a model of insomnia in the first place? Surely if you have it you have it, according to the diagnostic algorithm (see page 33), and there is no point trying to figure out why it happened?

The reason I always talk about Professor Spielman's model is that it tells an important story and it provides an insight as to why, later on during the course, I will be asking you to do certain things. Additionally, I feel that this is a really good way of looking at what makes you vulnerable to getting insomnia and, as such, it will aid in preventing the problem happening again when you have completed the course (see Day 7 – Maintaining Success and Relapse Prevention, page 157).

As we can see from my deconstructed version of Professor Spielman's model below (i), each of us has an 'insomnia threshold' whereby once that threshold is reached, or surpassed, the result will be the experiencing of the symptoms of insomnia (difficulty getting off to sleep, staying asleep and/or early morning awakening). Moreover, each of us has what Professor Spielman describes as a level of Predisposition to insomnia. What this means is that some of us are more vulnerable to insomnia than others. Where Professor Spielman talked about predisposition in terms of differences in gene expression and biology or certain personality characteristics, such as having an anxious or perfectionistic personality, I suggest, and the research confirms, that there are additional factors that make some of us more prone to insomnia than others. For example, we know that having had insomnia in the past makes you more vulnerable to develop insomnia in the future, as does getting older and being an evening-oriented person. I also believe that certain long-standing situations, such as caregiving, a history of shift work or having a chronic illness (physical or psychological), can also increase the risk of developing insomnia in the future.

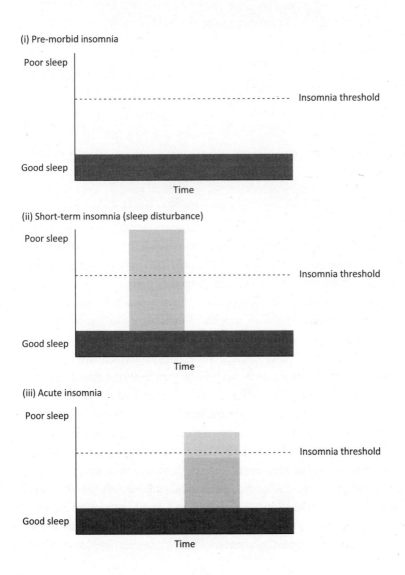

(i) Pre-morbid insomnia

Poor sleep

---------------------------------- Insomnia threshold

Good sleep

Time

(ii) Short-term insomnia (sleep disturbance)

Poor sleep

---------------------------------- Insomnia threshold

Good sleep

Time

(iii) Acute insomnia

Poor sleep

---------------------------------- Insomnia threshold

Good sleep

Time

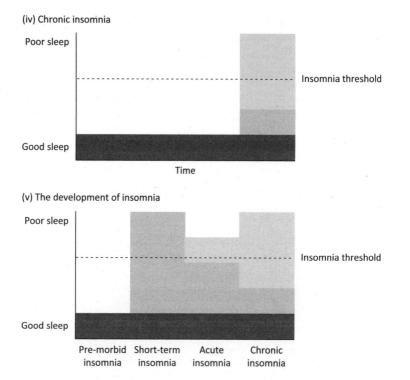

According to Professor Spielman (ii), something occurs (a Precipitating event) which, by the very nature of being stressful, pushes the individual over the insomnia threshold (into short-term insomnia or, as I like to call it, a sleep disturbance). Professor Spielman talked about precipitating factors as major life events (for example, divorce, bereavement, the onset of an illness, a new job, a new baby). In essence, the event has triggered the 'fight-or-flight' response and the body's natural reaction, due largely to the increase in stress-hormone production, is to reduce the amount of time you can sleep, presumably so you have more time to manage the current crisis.

That said, it stands to reason that, if you have more of a vulnerability to insomnia, what pushes you over the threshold does not necessarily have to be a major life event but perhaps a series of smaller irritations, a change in sleep environment or even the anticipation that something demanding or stressful is likely to happen. Over time (iii), the stress starts to reduce as the individual begins to manage or cope with the situation. Even if the situation, event or irritations continue, the stress response should reduce naturally as the body cannot maintain this 'heightened state of alertness' response for very long (remember the sleep homeostat needs to be reset or microsleeps will start to occur – see page 14).

This is the point at which Professor Spielman introduced the third and final 'P' – Perpetuating factors. He believed that, although the stress that caused the initial sleep disturbance diminishes somewhat, the insomnia begins to develop independently (acute insomnia), largely owing to the things we do to try to compensate for the reduced amount of sleep that we have been getting. These activities usually include changes to both daytime (for example, drinking more coffee to stay alert in the day) and night-time (going to bed early in search of lost sleep) routines and behaviours. Added to that the poor sleep has now become the focus of the stress, instead of what stressed us out in the first place, and we also begin to worry about the consequences of poor sleep on our day-to-day lives.

Eventually (iv), the impact of the initial trigger (precipitating factor) is negligible but the insomnia now exists in its own right, fuelled by increasingly complex behaviours, adopted in an attempt to get more sleep, and worries about the long-term consequences of having insomnia. By this time we become overly preoccupied with our sleep – ask any normal sleeper how they sleep and the response you will usually get is 'I don't know I just do it … it just happens', whereas someone with insomnia will probably have a lot more to say on the subject – and we become stuck in a vicious cycle of insomnia.

The main point to take away here is that it is not the event, be it a major life event or accumulation of irritations and hassles, that maintains the insomnia, it is largely the habits, rituals, behaviours and thoughts that we have developed to cope with, or compensate for, the initial sleep disturbance that serve to maintain the insomnia. Remember earlier when I talked about cognition and behaviour in relation to CBT-I (page 5)? This is essentially it: CBT-I is there to help you manage all of the rituals, habits, behaviours, worries and thoughts that are now feeding your insomnia. Hence why I believe that in most cases you can fix the problem yourself, using this course, and why I agreed to write this book in the first place.

How Do Perpetuating Factors Maintain Insomnia?

It is one thing to suggest that our own actions and thoughts, in the face of a period of sleep disturbance, can serve to maintain the insomnia through its acute phase and beyond but it is worth discussing how this actually happens.

Here I will deal with the most commonly seen perpetuating factor – excessive time in bed – and outline how this actually can maintain insomnia. Before that, I would like to make it clear that spending extra time in bed, in the face of an initial sleep disturbance or acute insomnia, seems like a logical, practical and rational thing to do, so I never blame people for doing this.

Several years ago, my friend and colleague, Dr Donn Posner, provided me with the most elegant description of what happens to our sleep when we spend excessive time in bed. Donn is, in my opinion, the best Cognitive Behaviour Therapy for Insomnia (CBT-I) therapist and supervisor I have ever met and I use his description every time I am either seeing an individual with insomnia or teaching a student or trainee how to do CBT-I.

Firstly, imagine a piece of pizza dough, pastry or such like. Let's say that this dough, fresh out of the packet or the can, represents how much time you should be spending in bed because of your biological sleep need. Now, I want you to imagine getting a knife and slicing several thin lines, say five or so, evenly across the pastry – almost as if you were going to make garlic bread with the dough. If you want to actually do this on a piece of dough or pastry, rather than simply imagining it, go for it – it actually helps make the point much clearer.

These lines you have cut represent the end of each sleep cycle throughout the night when we are most vulnerable to waking up. As I said earlier, after a short period of sleep disturbance, we tend to compensate by spending more time in bed either by going to bed early and/or having a lie-in. So, stretch out the dough, let's say by 1½ –2 inches, each side, to represent this increased amount of time in bed. Also, bear in mind that your biological sleep need has not changed, as it cannot change that much and certainly not that quickly.

If you now look at the dough you will notice two things: firstly, the dough has become quite thin, almost transparent, in places and may now have holes in it and, secondly, those thin lines you cut have expanded, becoming much bigger. This is what happens to your sleep when you extend your time in bed. Your sleep has now become thin (lighter) with holes in it (awakenings in the night) and those thin lines that you cut (potential vulnerabilities for an awakening at the end of each sleep cycle) have now greatly increased.

What we tend to see happen next is that the response to this period of acute insomnia (maintained by the extended time in bed, amongst other things) is to spend even more time in bed to make up for the lost sleep, waiting for the sandman to come, and so a vicious cycle of poor sleep ensues into the chronic phase of insomnia and beyond.

What Does Insomnia Actually Look Like?

We have looked at the diagnosis of insomnia and shown, using Professor Spielman's model, how insomnia develops and can be maintained, but how does this information actually translate into the experience of insomnia? Here, I am going to use a case study to demonstrate.

Case Study: Lydia

Lydia is a 42-year-old woman. She is a principal social worker with over 25 years of social work experience. She is divorced and has three grown-up children. None of the children live at home but she does have a significant other. She describes herself as reasonably healthy, with only minor ailments (coughs, colds, etc.) periodically affecting her. She is on no prescription medications and has no history of any major physical or psychological illnesses although she reported that her day-to-day stress level is 'at a constant high'. I have already assessed Lydia for other sleep disorders, with the help of her significant other, and she appears not to have any other sleep issues or disorders. She has an intermediate chronotype, as does her significant other. In terms of her past sleep history, she describes herself as 'always being a light sleeper', but has never regarded herself as having a sleep problem till now. She also describes herself as 'a bit of a worrier', especially when it comes to her work and the people she manages.

At our first meeting Lydia told me that she ' ... has lost sleep'. When prompted, she stated: 'I have lost it [sleep], the ability to do it ... manage it, to hold on to it ... it's just not there when I really need it anymore.' I asked Lydia when the problem started and if she could recall a specific event or series of events that sparked the period of poor sleep. She responded by saying that she has had the problem (insomnia) for about two years and it started around the time of a restructure at work in which her team was drastically cut, although the amount of casework they shared remained the same. I asked Lydia to describe the problem she was having with her sleep and she told me that the predominant issue was one of getting off to sleep, with it regularly taking her 90 minutes, or more, to get off to sleep at night. When asked how frequently this happens in a 'typical' week she said 'most nights'. She also reported being awake in the night for about 10–15 minutes but that was rare – once or twice a month. I then asked Lydia whether she felt the sleep problem was impacting on her day-to-day life. She responded by saying that everything feels 'slowed down', that she can't think as fast as she used to and she finds herself losing her temper with her work colleagues, but mainly with herself, far too easily. She believes that this is because she is not sleeping and, ultimately, it is affecting her performance at work as she keeps forgetting to do things.

I then asked Lydia to describe a 'typical' workday for me. Lydia reported getting up at 6am (almost always feeling tired), showering, getting ready for work and then having breakfast. She usually leaves the house at around 7.15 to get to work (drives) for 8. She finishes her office work around 6pm and would get home about 6.45–7pm, depending on traffic. She would continue to 'catch up' on work till about 9pm, when she and her partner would have dinner and watch some television. Lydia reported that usually she would fall asleep, albeit briefly, on the sofa and then, realising she was ready for sleep, 'drag' herself off to bed anywhere between 10 and 10.30pm. However, she then described her experience of going to bed ' ... so I know I am tired as I just fell asleep on the sofa ... so I head off to bed as quick as I can. It's like clockwork ... I make it upstairs ... yawning ... and go to brush my teeth. As soon as I start brushing I feel myself waking up! Becoming more alert ... By the time I get into bed, I am fully awake and I just know what is going to happen next ... I am going to lie there and then start thinking about tomorrow, wondering what I have to do next and then worrying about all the decisions I made today and what I forgot to do ... The more I tell myself to stop it [thinking about things] and focus on getting to sleep the more it [thinking] happens and then I can't seem to stop.'

I then asked Lydia whether her sleep pattern was any different on non-work days. She responded that she would probably go to bed later at the weekend (10.30–11pm) and she would stay in bed till about 8.30–9.30 the next morning. I next asked Lydia what she does, throughout the day and night, to manage her sleep problem and her feelings of sleepiness in the daytime. She responded that she would 'do all kinds of weird and wonderful stuff', including drinking lots of energy drinks, especially in the late afternoon when she felt particularly drained, using antihistamines (only occasionally) to help her sleep at night, reading or watching TV in bed to pass the time and trying to get an early night whenever she could.

Finally, I asked Lydia about her thoughts and beliefs about sleep – how much sleep she feels she needs to function properly, what she believes the consequences (short term and long term) are for her from not getting the right amount of sleep, how often she thinks about her sleep during the day and the extent to which she feels that her sleep problem is permanent. With respect to these last questions, Lydia felt that she probably needed at least 7–8 hours of sleep a night to function properly, that in the short term her poor sleep has already resulted in poor performance at work (physically and psychologically) but in the long term her current sleep problems were likely to make her very, very ill. She also reported that she believed her sleep problems to be permanent and that she found herself dwelling on the topic of her own sleep 'almost all the time' during the day.

This is a typical, albeit uncomplicated, case of insomnia and Lydia was definitely a candidate for CBT-I (and she did exceptionally well, I am pleased to say). You can see from Lydia's experiences, that she meets all the six criteria for insomnia (see page 33) and a pattern of predisposing (anxious personality and history of being a light sleeper), precipitating (the work restructuring two years ago and the constant stress of work) and perpetuating factors – both behavioural (excessive amounts of time in bed not sleeping, variable sleep schedules, reading/watching TV in bed, using caffeinated drinks to stay awake and using antihistamines to help her sleep) and cognitive (worrying in bed, dysfunctional beliefs about sleep, sleep-related catastrophic thinking – see page 143 for more on this last factor).

However, Lydia's story gives us an insight into an additional perpetuating factor that we have not yet discussed – sleep effort. As we can see, Lydia talks about 'focusing on getting to sleep' when she is in bed. As we mentioned earlier, normal sleepers, when asked, will not be able to tell you how they do it (sleep) and are very unlikely to say that they have to try or do anything specific to achieve sleep.

The term 'sleep effort' comes from Professor Colin Espie. He suggests that trying to achieve a goal that is not under your direct control (in this case, sleeping) is likely to be ineffective but, even more problematic, is the fact that the more you try to achieve the goal, the more you will become overly focused on what is becoming an unachievable goal, become anxious, frustrated and worried at not achieving the goal, and become physically and psychologically tense as a result of that increased attention to the goal. These three states are clearly incompatible with sleep, thus the effort used to sleep serves to perpetuate the insomnia through increased levels of arousal (physical tension and mental alertness) at night. As you will see in Part 2, we have a specific technique that directly addresses sleep effort as well as a few techniques that will indirectly stop you from effortful sleeping.

Conditioned Responses and Conditioned Arousal

The next concept I am going to discuss is related to how someone with insomnia develops an overly negative evaluation of their bedroom and bedtime routine – through a conditioned response. Here, I am going to give an example of how conditioning works, using my favourite analogy, food, again, before discussing how this translates to conditioned arousal.

I work from home sometimes and, when I work from home, I usually work at my desk in my office (sounds fancier than it is). A little while ago, I was having repairs done to the ceiling in my office so I decided to work in the dining room instead (it has a big table and I tend to be quite messy and spread papers everywhere). Soon I began to notice that I was putting on weight. Why did this happen? Because the dining table is where I always eat when I am at home, I found myself snacking more while I was working. The dining room and the dining table, in particular, for me, is a stimulus, which now (after a period of eating in the dining room and nowhere else in the house) is associated with another specific, albeit biological, stimulus (to eat). However, the conditioned response part was that I was getting hungrier when I was working in the dining room because I unconsciously expected to be in there to eat.

When I moved back into my office, I noticed something else: I began to regularly eat snacks in my office. The pairing of these two stimuli – working and snacking, which I had been doing in the dining room frequently over the previous couple of weeks – had transferred from the dining room to my newly repaired office. That was an extension of that initial conditioned behaviour. But how does that relate to conditioned arousal?

Conditioned arousal incorporates a conditioned response, but the response is more of a visceral/emotional reaction to the pairing of the stimuli. Although we can see clearly the factors that perpetuate insomnia in Lydia's case (including sleep effort), one of the main overarching issues here, which needed some consideration in her treatment, is her conditioned arousal to the bed and bedtime routine which, as we saw on page 40, is a significant feature of Psychophysiologic Insomnia.

In Lydia's case, she describes this as the feeling she gets of becoming fully awake when she brushes her teeth, as part of her normal sleep routine. Others have described this experience as 'all the lights coming on in my head', 'a flick of a switch' or 'a silent alarm going off' when reaching the bedroom at night. Additionally, when you ask people with insomnia how they feel about their bed, many will respond with comments like '[my bed is like] a bed of ... thorns ... nails ... thistles'. Together, these narratives point to someone who no longer sees sleep as a pleasurable, or even a neutral, activity but as a combative or aversive experience. The initial pairing of their bedroom/bed and poor sleep, during the acute phase of insomnia will, given enough time, result in an automatic association between two previously unconditioned stimuli (their bed and them being awake). With enough pairings, the stimulus itself – seeing their bed or even the thought of it – is enough to evoke a conditioned arousal response, either physical (increased tension) or psychological (fear and anxiety at the thought of not sleeping), which can arouse us and keep us awake at night. Again, physical tension, fear and anxiety are not compatible with going to sleep or staying asleep and so the chances of not getting a good night's sleep increase and add weight to the vicious cycle of insomnia.

When I am looking to see if an individual with insomnia has conditioned arousal, in addition to listening to how they describe their bed and their pre-sleep routine, I will usually ask them how they sleep for the first night in an unfamiliar environment (such as a hotel, or a friend's or relative's house). If they respond by saying that they would generally sleep a bit better, that is reasonably good evidence that there is some degree of conditioned arousal to their bedroom that needs to be addressed. However, I tend to see evidence of conditioned arousal most clearly when someone with insomnia sleeps in my laboratory, which is rare but not unheard of. On the first night in the laboratory, a large percentage of people with insomnia (particularly those with Psychophysiologic Insomnia) tend to sleep much better than they do at home, which can be a little disconcerting for them in the morning. This phenomenon is quite common and is referred to as the Reverse First Night Effect (RFNE). Unfortunately, this phenomenon appears to last just one night, otherwise it would be a very easy and effective treatment option, and the individual with insomnia will most likely sleep poorly in the lab on the second night and thereafter.

Cortical Arousal

The last concept that I want to discuss in this section is cortical arousal. Again, you can see how this manifests in Lydia's story when she describes herself as always being a 'light sleeper'. This is a common phenomenon for lots of people with insomnia, either throughout their entire lives or at some specific time point in their life (for example, it can occur more frequently in the third trimester of pregnancy).

Although mainly a theoretical concept at present (the topic has not been systematically researched in insomnia, although I should note the excellent work being done by Professor Celyne Bastien, Professor Dan Buysse and Dr Michael Perlis), it does possess a certain degree of logic, especially when listening to the experiences of people with insomnia. What we believe is that, the brain, for whatever reason, remains in a state of heightened alertness and vigilance even when the physical body is at rest (sleep). As such, in this state we still have the potential to attend and monitor the external environment (for example, a thunderstorm) and/or our internal sensations (aches and pains) while we are sleeping and we store some of this information in our memories. In the morning we can recall some of this information (we may not precisely know what it was that we heard or felt) and interpret this as a sign of being awake during the night. In its extreme form this may well explain the existence of Paradoxical Insomnia, although it is likely that we all have a certain degree of cortical arousal at night and this will change, depending upon certain circumstances (illness, pregnancy, stress). The difficulty is that not all patients with insomnia demonstrate high levels of cortical arousal (at the moment we measure this through high-frequency brainwave activity) and so it is not necessarily a defining characteristic of all insomnia. It is most likely best classified as a vulnerability factor (predisposing factor) if it has been there since birth or as a precipitating factor if levels of cortical arousal increase when we are stressed or under unusual circumstances.

Create Your Personal Version of Professor Spielman's Model of Insomnia

I am sure you will be pleased to know that we have finished with models and theories of insomnia, at least for now.

The first activity that I would like you to do is personalise your own version of Professor Spielman's model. Using the template below, identify any predisposing factors that you feel make you, as a person, particularly vulnerable to insomnia. I have provided an example to help guide you when you are completing your personalised version. Then identify the precipitating event, or series of events or hassles, that led to the start of your insomnia (remember – the event does not always have to be a negative event, just something that challenged your existing resources such as planning a wedding, a promotion at work, an exam). Now, and most importantly, list all the behaviours you currently engage in to compensate for your insomnia or ways in which you try to get more sleep and all the thoughts, feelings and beliefs that you have about your sleep. Keep this safe throughout the course, as you will probably add to it as we go along. We will refer to it when we talk about Relapse Prevention (see page 157).

Predisposing Factors	Precipitating Factors	Perpetuating Factors
Anxious personality	Divorce	Drink coffee throughout the day
Mother had insomnia	Had to sell house	Worry
I have had insomnia in the past	Had to move	Go to bed early
		No regular sleep pattern
		Watch TV in my bedroom
		Nap at weekends
		I think I need 8 hours sleep to function
		Can't stop thinking about sleep
		I am not productive at work

Predisposing Factors	Precipitating Factors	Perpetuating Factors

Before You Start the Course

Am I a Candidate for the Course?

If we have got this far together, you have met all six criteria for insomnia and don't appear to have Paradoxical Insomnia so we can go forward with the algorithm to determine whether you are a candidate for the course. Remember that the insomnia must have been present for at least two weeks before you can start the course.

The next thing we need to discuss is if the course is right for you, right now. The first thing to say about that is that although there may be reasons (discussed below) that may prevent you from doing the full course at this time, in most cases some consideration or management of those circumstances will not prevent you from doing the course, or at least a revised version of it, at some point in the future.

There are, however, some illnesses and conditions where the course is NOT appropriate for you and in these instances I would recommend seeing a Behavioural Sleep Medicine specialist for individual face-to-face treatment for your insomnia. Why? Because it is my belief that, under these special circumstances, you may need more guidance and support than this fabulous book can offer on its own and so face-to-face treatment would ensure the best outcome possible for you. One of these conditions, which I don't talk about in the algorithm but is important to mention, is people with an Intellectual Disability. The main reason I feel additional face-to-face support may be needed is because of the high levels of overlap between insomnia and complex circadian rhythm disorders in this group of people. As such, a careful assessment of what needs to be addressed first and how is, in my opinion, very important.

Using the Algorithm

We will go through the algorithm one step at a time to determine whether this course is right for you, right now. What you will probably notice first is that there are three possible outcomes following your progression through the algorithm. The first, where the course is NOT indicated, the second where the course is NOT indicated AT THIS TIME, which suggests something should be attended to before you start the course, and the third, which is where the full course IS indicated and you can progress to the pre-planning stage. You need to work through this next section carefully and only when you have reached the end and the course IS indicated should you do the course.

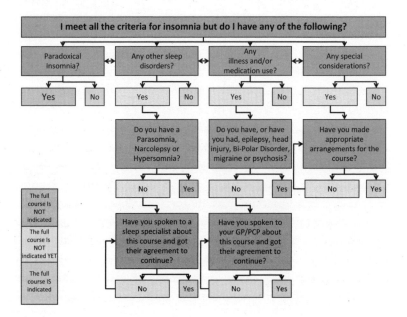

So, assuming that you meet all the criteria for insomnia, including having it for at least two weeks, and do not meet criteria for Paradoxical Insomnia, we need to look at whether any pre-existing illness, disorder or circumstance could make parts of the course unsuitable for you. We know from hundreds of studies that CBT-I is, in the main, safe, effective and durable. In fact, CBT-I has been used successfully in a range of patient groups ranging from those with depression or anxiety disorders through to those with various types of cancer, coronary heart disease and fibromyalgia. Additionally, many studies have demonstrated that CBT-I is suitable for all adult age groups, including older adults. Our main consideration here is the, albeit temporary, increased amounts of daytime sleepiness caused when you undertake the sleep rescheduling (see page 107) and stimulus control (see page 119) aspects of the course and the additional impact that increased sleepiness may have on any existing condition that you might have.

The other main consideration is the cognitive distraction techniques (see page 137), which have the potential to make the symptoms of some specific illnesses worse. We will address whether you are a candidate for the course by examining three areas – other sleep problems, illnesses and medications, and roles and responsibilities.

AN IMPORTANT NOTE BEFORE YOU BEGIN THE COURSE

What I would stress is that, before you begin the course, if you are seeing a healthcare professional such as a GP/PCP, consultant or specialist because of any on-going physical or psychological illness, sleep disorder or medication, discuss this course with your healthcare provider and specifically find out whether any existing issues would prohibit you from doing the full course. While this is happening what you can do is examine and manage your sleep hygiene (see page 86) and keep a Pre-course Sleep Diary (see page 94).

Other Sleep Disorders

It is important to note that you can have two or more sleep disorders at the same time, so having another sleep disorder does not necessarily mean that you cannot have insomnia and vice versa. There are a wide range of other sleep disorders out there, some of which suggest caution and some for which a form of management is needed before you can do the full course.

Traditionally, sleep disorders were defined under two main headings – Disorders of Initiating and Maintaining Sleep (DIMS) and Disorders of Excessive daytime Sleepiness/Somnolence (DOES). This way of classifying sleep disorders, although rarely used these days, is helpful to us in the sense that many DIMS may in fact look a lot like insomnia but it may not always be the case, whereas DOES do not tend to look that much like insomnia but they can complicate the management of it.

Here, I will cover the most commonly encountered DIMS and DOES and outline whether or not the course is suitable in each case or what you will need to do before starting the course.

Where DIMS, naturally, would cover insomnia, they also cover Circadian Rhythm Disorders.

Circadian Rhythm Disorders

Broadly, Circadian Rhythm Disorders (CRDs) cover any circumstance or condition that results in a mismatch between the timing of the biological sleep/wake circadian rhythm and the timing of the external world (for example, the jet lag associated with air travel). This can be caused by situational events such as doing rotating shift work over a long period of time or a rapid change in time zone (trans-meridian flight), a physical condition that makes you more vulnerable (for example, blindness) or even a normal maturation event, such as puberty. The main difference between those with insomnia and those with a CRD is that, given the opportunity to sleep whenever they liked (*ad libitum*), those with CRDs are likely to be able to get off to sleep easily, stay asleep during the night and generally feel rested on waking, whereas those with insomnia would still not be able to get off to sleep or stay asleep.

Is having a CRD a reason to not do the full course (assuming you meet all the criteria for insomnia)? Not necessarily although, if you have an untreated or severe CRD, the course will be much, much harder to tolerate. As such, I feel it is important to see a Behavioural Sleep Medicine specialist in order to assess and, if necessary, address the CRD before you begin as this will make the course a much more manageable experience and, ultimately, give you better results. That said, there are a few occasions where a CRD can look a lot like insomnia but may in fact 'better explain' the insomnia (see What Do We Classify As Insomnia? on page 33). If the sleep/wake circadian cycle is advanced, it may look like late insomnia and if the sleep/wake circadian cycle is delayed, it may look like initial insomnia. This is another reason to get a CRD checked out before you start the course.

Disorders of Excessive Daytime Sleepiness

Disorders of Excessive Daytime Sleepiness (DOES), on the other hand, cover a range of sleep disorders including Restless Legs Syndrome, Periodic Limb Movement Disorders, Parasomnias, Obstructive Sleep Apnea (OSA), Narcolepsy and Hypersomnia or hypersomnolence disorders.

Obstructive Sleep Apnea

OSA is part of a larger family of sleep-related breathing disorders. An apnea event occurs when there is a partial or total blockage in the upper airway, for at least 10 seconds, during the night.

This blockage, usually caused by a loss of muscle tension around the airway (soft palate), results in bursts of shallow breathing accompanied by loud snoring, then in some cases a total, albeit relatively brief, period where you stop breathing altogether. In this case, levels of carbon dioxide in your blood increase as the levels of oxygen in the blood decrease. The diaphragm and chest muscles try to get air back into the lungs and signal the brain to wake up in order to tense the muscles in the soft palate and re-open the airway. The result will be a loud snort, gasp or choking noise (not to be confused with loud snoring which is evidence of the airway being partially obstructed but not closed) from the individual as their breathing resumes.

As you would expect, this increased effort to breathe will create an arousal, which interrupts sleep, although the individual is not always aware of the arousal. This results in the sleep stage that we were in becoming fragmented. We all experience apnea events at some point, in fact more frequently than you would think, and there are many situations that increase the number of apnea events we may experience in a night, for example when we have a head cold or a respiratory infection. Additionally, many substances such as alcohol, tobacco and some prescribed sleep medications for insomnia can also increase the frequency of apnea (total closures) or hypopnea (partial closures) events during the night.

However, the diagnosis of Obstructive Sleep Apnea is determined on the basis of how many apnea/hypopnea events occur per hour of sleep. Below 5 events per hour of sleep is considered normal, more than 5 but fewer than 15 events per hour of sleep is considered mild OSA, more than 15 but fewer than 30 is considered moderate OSA and over 30 events per hour of sleep (1 every 2 minutes) is considered severe OSA.

In the case of OSA, the individual is likely to report very unrefreshing sleep and feel excessively sleepy during the day, perhaps even needing a nap or dozing off unintentionally on occasion, but they are unlikely to pinpoint the reason for this excessive lethargy. Interestingly, OSA is generally a partner-reported condition in that the partner is woken by a pattern of loud snoring, a period of silence and then a loud gasp for breath. Other, less commonly reported symptoms, which may be helpful to identify OSA if you don't have a bed-partner, in addition to the unexplainable excessive daytime sleepiness, are morning headaches, a dry mouth or sore throat in the morning, increased blood pressure, unexplained weight gain, and/or frequent episodes of heartburn.

Unfortunately, as that list could also explain a whole host of other illnesses, you will need to discuss these symptoms with your GP/PCP and be tested for OSA. Contrary to popular belief, you don't have to be male, older and overweight to have OSA (although each of these three things increases the risk of you developing OSA). In fact, the most severe case I have ever witnessed was a young, slim woman.

So, is the full course right for you if you have OSA and insomnia? The answer is NO, not right now. The thing to do is get the OSA under control before you start the course as the mild sleep deprivation caused by the sleep rescheduling (see page 107) and stimulus control (see page 119) aspects of the course may increase the amount of daytime sleepiness that is already there, due to the OSA, making you more prone to accidents and mistakes.

The good news is that are some excellent treatment options out there for both mild/moderate and severe OSA and I would recommend asking for a referral to a specialist in respiratory medicine or Ear, Nose and Throat (ENT) medicine. I will discuss the treatment options for OSA on page 183. Once the OSA is under control and, if the insomnia remains, then the course will be fine to do in its entirety, as with CRDs and RLS. That said, I would probably discuss the course with your consultant before starting just to make sure you are good to go.

Narcolepsy

This is a neurological disorder whereby the affected individual experiences 'sleep attacks' (unintentional and uncontrollable episodes of falling asleep during the day). The main symptoms of Narcolepsy are excessive daytime sleepiness, temporary loss of voluntary muscle control (known as cataplexy), hallucinations and sleep paralysis (the inability to move on awakening). In most cases, Narcolepsy will be diagnosed by a neurologist who will use both a night-time polysomnography test and a series of daytime polysomnography tests (known as a Multiple Sleep Latency Test). In these instances, the diagnosis can be determined largely on how quickly you enter REM during these tests.

Can this course be beneficial for an individual with Narcolepsy? To be frank, there have been no studies to date, that I know of, that have examined the impact of a CBT-I framework (either the full six–eight-week programme or briefer forms such as this one) on people with Narcolepsy and what cognitive and behavioural advice there is for people with Narcolepsy tends to be opposite to what we would be doing in the course (for example, recommended short naps in the afternoons). So, at this time, I do NOT recommend the course for someone who has Narcolepsy even if they have insomnia alongside their Narcolepsy (which is more common than you would think). A neurologist will be able to diagnose your Narcolepsy and, if appropriate, work with you, alongside a Behavioural Sleep Medicine specialist, to help manage your insomnia.

Hypersomnia

The final DOES we will discuss is Hypersomnia. Hypersomnia is a broad category for a host of disorders that are all characterised by excessive daytime sleepiness. In many cases, another illness, disease or disorder can explain the hypersomnolence (for example, OSA or Narcolepsy) but in the case of Idiopathic Hypersomnia the excessive daytime sleepiness exists despite adequate sleep and individuals may need in excess of 10 hours of sleep a night. In light of this, Idiopathic Hypersomnia is not really likely to co-occur with insomnia and so the course would NOT be suitable.

Restless Legs Syndrome

Restless Legs Syndrome (RLS) or Willis-Ekbom Disease, as it is otherwise known, is a disorder characterised by an irresistible urge to move your legs, commonly accompanied by an uncomfortable, itchy, crawly sensation in the legs. These symptoms tend to worsen when you have been sitting still for some time (like on an aeroplane) or generally as the evening progresses. In most cases RLS is alleviated, albeit temporarily, by moving the afflicted area (in other words, by walking about). RLS can look a lot like a form of initial insomnia in that people who have RLS commonly report difficulties getting off to sleep but this is largely due to the sensations they are experiencing. In my experience, RLS, like CRDs, is one of those disorders that, in a few cases, can 'better explain' the insomnia.

One of the other things to mention about RLS is that we see quite high levels associated with pregnancy, heavy menstruation and/or poor diet. This is largely to do with low iron levels or the reduced capacity to bind to proteins (stay in the body) and, if you suspect you might have RLS for one of those reasons, consult your GP/PCP and ask for a ferritin blood test. If it is the case that your RLS is due to low iron or the capacity to bind iron then, once it is managed, the RLS should, in most cases, go away as should any difficulties getting off to sleep.

For those with RLS not due to low iron levels, a specialist in movement disorders (most likely a neurologist) will be able to help and the course is NOT suitable until the RLS is being managed (and, of course, if you still meet all the criteria for insomnia after successful management).

Periodic Limb Movement Disorder

Periodic Limb Movement Disorder (PLMD) is similar in some respects to RLS (in fact, around 80% of people with RLS also have PLMD) in that there is sometimes cramping or an uncomfortable sensation in the legs (although this can affect other limbs too), but PLMD can be a more painful experience than RLS. Additionally, it tends to occur when we are asleep, as opposed to RLS, and is associated with brief jerking movements during sleep. In this instance PLMD can look, at first glance, somewhat like a form of middle or late insomnia in that people with PLMD will report restless sleep and being unrefreshed on waking in the morning.

That said, many people with PLMD do not report actual awakenings in the night or the long periods of wakefulness during the night that characterise middle or late insomnia. Having PLMD should not prevent you from doing the full course if you have insomnia. In fact, there is evidence that CBT-I can actually help with the symptoms of PLMD, but it is always worth seeing a specialist in movement disorders or a Behavioural Sleep Medicine specialist if you suspect that you have PLMD, to get a proper assessment and management plan before starting the course.

Parasomnias

There is a wide variety of types of Parasomnias, including nightmares, night terrors, sleepwalking, bruxism (teeth grinding), confusional arousals, sleep paralysis and REM Behaviour Disorder (RBD). In essence, Parasomnias are associated with an arousal from REM sleep or a partial arousal from non-REM sleep. In the simplest terms, two states (wakefulness and a sleep stage) have collided, resulting in the individual performing actions that would not normally occur because the body should be in a state of partial or full paralysis. Similar to someone with PLMD, an individual with a Parasomnia may report restless sleep and being unrefreshed on waking, but is unlikely to recall actually being awake during the night.

However, unlike PLMD, I strongly recommend seeing a neurologist or Behavioural Sleep Medicine specialist for treatment and NOT undertaking the course if you have a Parasomnia, even if you meet all the criteria for insomnia. The difficulty is that the mild sleep deprivation caused by sleep rescheduling (see page 107) and stimulus control (see page 119) can increase the likelihood of a Parasomnia episode. Managing sleep hygiene (see page 86) would be a suitable start, alongside keeping the Pre-course Sleep Diary, while you are waiting for an appointment.

To Sum Up

So, to summarise, if you have a CRD or PLMD I recommend that you can do the full course but it would be helpful to have the CRD or PLMD successfully managed beforehand, just to make the course more tolerable. If you have RLS or OSA I strongly recommend you be assessed and treated before you start the course, to make sure the RLS or OSA is not explaining your symptoms, and if you have a Parasomnia, Narcolepsy or Hypersomnia the course is NOT right for you and you should discuss treatment options with a Behavioural Sleep Medicine specialist or other healthcare professional.

Illnesses and Medications

I have already mentioned that CBT-I has been successful for individuals with a range of physical and psychological illnesses, but are there any illnesses where this course may not be appropriate?

There are two parts to this answer – any illness or condition that is not being managed can be a problem and any illness or condition where even a mild form of sleep deprivation exists may make the illness worse.

In terms of the first part of the answer, this goes back to the diagnosis of insomnia and the sixth criterion (see page 39) that the insomnia should not be 'adequately explained' by another illness or condition. If, after appropriate management of the other condition (in other words, when the other condition is stable), the insomnia remains, then the course should be fine to do. However, as I have said before, I strongly advise anyone with an illness, condition or disorder to discuss the course with his or her GP/PCP prior to starting, irrespective of whether it is under control, or not, just to be sure.

There are six specific conditions for which this course is NOT appropriate at all: Bi-Polar Disorder, psychosis, epilepsy or if you have a history of seizures, Post Traumatic Stress Disorder (PTSD), migraine or head injury.

In each of these cases the mild sleep deprivation from the sleep rescheduling (see page 107) and stimulus control (see page 119) can cause the existing condition to worsen quite quickly. Moreover, the strategies covered under the technique of Cognitive Distraction (see page 137) could also be problematic and trigger a worsening in symptoms, especially in the case of PTSD, psychosis or migraine. That is not to say that CBT-I would not work with an individual who has any one of these conditions (in fact, there is evidence that it does help in each case), but this is where individual monitoring and constant support by a healthcare professional, preferably a healthcare professional with a knowledge of behavioural sleep medicine, is an absolute necessity.

What About Medications?

Most medications that cross the blood–brain barrier affect sleep in one way or another. Some can disrupt sleep, while others can make us more drowsy, sleepy or fatigued during the day. Here, there are three questions to take to your GP/PCP:

1. Are there any medications that I am currently taking that could be affecting my sleep?
2. Is there any combination of medications that I am currently taking that could be affecting my sleep?
3. Are there any medications that I am currently taking that would be affected by a brief period of mild sleep deprivation?

If the answer to those three questions is negative then, as long as you meet all the criteria for insomnia, you are good to go with the full course. If there are medications that may be affecting your sleep or, indeed, will be affected by a brief period of mild sleep deprivation then it may be worth exploring, with your GP/PCP, alternative medications or countermeasures that you can put into place during the course that will minimise the impact of the medication.

Recovery

The last thing I want to talk about in this section is recovery. While there are a few studies that have used CBT-I in individuals recovering from substance abuse, with some good outcomes, there are additional challenges for this group of people that should be taken into account.

While I am not saying that the course is not right for you, if this is the case, I think the main thing to be mindful of is how far into your recovery period you are. We know, for example, that long-term use of substances such as alcohol or cocaine tends to change the architecture of our sleep quite a bit. So sleep tends to get a bit messy during the early part of recovery, as we are trying to re-establish, both biologically and socially, new sleep routines and patterns. Adding on an, albeit brief, period of mild sleep deprivation would not be good at that time and so I would suggest that you should be in recovery for at least 18 months before you do the course and, even then, you should discuss the course with your GP/PCP or consultant before starting.

What happens if you have a bad case of insomnia during that time? Here again is a situation that I believe needs some extra support and guidance and a referral to a Behavioural Sleep Medicine specialist, for individual face-to-face treatment, would be the best way forward.

So, to summarise this section, the course should be discussed if you have any illness, condition or medication use (other than the six conditions mentioned above, where the course is not appropriate at all) with your GP/PCP before you begin. If the illness is under control, the medications you are taking are not going to be affected by a brief period of mild sleep deprivation and your GP/PCP can see no reason preventing you from doing the course then the full course is indicated. Finally, if you are in recovery, the full course is indicated as long as you have been in recovery for at least 18 months and discussed the course with your GP/PCP.

Roles and Responsibilities

Here, I am mainly going to focus on occupations where I feel extra caution is required. I am not suggesting that the full course is not appropriate, just that extra care and attention and perhaps some extra planning should be put in place before starting.

I am mainly talking about occupations whereby even a small, albeit brief, amount of sleep deprivation can potentially cause harm to the self or to others. So we are talking about any job that involves a great deal of driving (for example, long-distance lorry drivers, bus drivers, taxi drivers, train drivers), requires heightened levels of attention and vigilance for long periods of time (for example, air-traffic controllers) or sustained periods of concentration (for example, surgeons).

In these instances rescheduling work commitments for the week would be a really good way forward or, if that is not possible, perhaps start the course at the weekend (or on equivalent days off) when the majority of the mild sleep deprivation will occur and so the course will be more manageable.

Also there is the rather overlooked occupation of caregiving, be that for children, older adults or an individual with an illness or condition who needs support. And yes, I do classify anyone, paid or otherwise, who is giving care to another as a caregiver. Again, I would recommend enlisting some extra support, if at all possible and appropriate, while doing the course. My concern here is the temporary impact that the mild sleep deprivation can have on your mood and ability to cope with what may already be a stressful occupation and/or stressful set of life circumstances.

Children

Is the course suitable for children? To my knowledge, CBT-I has never been used with children, the reason being that, if they suffer from insomnia, it is generally not quite the same thing as adult insomnia. As such CBT-I, and indeed this course, are NOT suitable for children (those under 18 years old) and may do more harm than good because of the sleep rescheduling and stimulus control aspects, which could interfere with 'normal' development. In a case of childhood insomnia I would always recommend seeking out a Paediatric Sleep Medicine specialist for a thorough investigation.

Older Adults

Finally, let's talk about older adults. There are a vast number of published studies that demonstrate that full CBT-I and briefer versions, such as this one, are suitable and work just as well for older adults as they do for younger adults. That said, I personally feel that we need to explore one specific issue when dealing with treating insomnia in an older adult, namely the risk of falling.

While falls can happen to everyone, the increased levels of illness and medication use make older adults particularly vulnerable to falls. If you have had a fall in the past, which in itself increases the risk of a future fall, or you feel that you may be more vulnerable to falling, for whatever reason, I recommend that you read the special note on Alternatives to Leaving the Bed and Alternatives to Leaving the Bedroom on page 127. Apart from that, the rest of the course should be just fine.

Shift Work

Is the course appropriate for someone who does shift work? The answer to this is yes and no, depending on the shifts' timing and the frequency with which your shift patterns change.

For someone who does shift work where the actual hours of the shift do not change, there should be no significant problem in doing the full course. That said, be more mindful about the mild sleep deprivation from the sleep rescheduling (see page 107) and stimulus control (see page 119), as a lot of people who do night shift work are already a bit sleep deprived as it is harder, logistically and biologically, to sleep during the daytime due to the sleep wake circadian rhythm.

If, however, you do rotating shifts, this will be a problem and I would NOT recommend you doing the full course while you are doing these shifts. The reason for this is that, as you will see later, one of the most important parts of the course is determining your personal sleep plan and sticking to it every day. This is going to be impossible if you are doing rotating shift work, as you are unlikely to be able to stick to your new sleep pattern because of your changing work commitments. In the case of rotating shift work, what I would suggest here is going to see a Behavioural Sleep Medicine specialist to determine whether you have a Circadian Rhythm Disorder that is masking as insomnia before even starting the course. If there is no CRD, my advice would be to do everything EXCEPT sleep rescheduling and stimulus control and then perhaps enlist an experienced Behavioural Sleep Medicine specialist to help you create an individualised plan to tackle the sleep rescheduling and stimulus control aspects of the course.

So, to summarise, you need to take account of how a brief period of mild sleep deprivation will affect the roles and responsibilities that you have in your life. If you are in an occupation where extra precautions should be taken and/or extra support should be enlisted, then, as long as you have put some safeguards in place, the full course should be fine to do. The main consideration is making sure you and others are kept safe during the course. In the most broad sense, I will refer to guidelines that are issued every day with the thousands of medications that have the potential to make us sleepy or drowsy during the day: if you feel sleepy or drowsy 'do not drive or operate tools or machinery'.

Pre-planning

While it would be great to just get going on the course now, a little bit of pre-planning, in my experience, goes a long way. In fact, it will increase your chances of following through with the course and seeing its full benefits. What do I mean by pre-planning? I will talk about it in two main areas – pre-planning for you and preparing others.

Pre-planning for You

It is probably the case that you could find several reasons why you should start the course at another time, especially after what I have just said about those occupations where extra consideration and precautions are needed. So you may be asking: should I do it during a less stressful time at work? Should I wait to start it while I am on vacation? Should I wait until things have calmed down a little? Should I wait and start the course when the kids are on holiday?

I am going to challenge those concerns and say that, if you have got to this point and everything is good to go, including making extra provisions if you need to, you can start preparing for the course at any time but this should preferably be done sooner rather than later. My reasons for this are two-fold:

1. We all have a habit of putting things off and the longer we put things off the more likely we will not even start them in the first place. Presumably you got, or were given, this book for a reason. If you satisfy all the criteria for insomnia and there are no outstanding problems or issues that need some extra attention (see Am I a Candidate for the Course? on page 61), then there should be nothing stopping you from starting planning for the course right away.

2. By the end of the course I want you to be able to sleep normally in any environment, under any 'normal' circumstances. If you were to start the course after taking lots and lots of extra precautions (for example, sending the kids to stay with relatives or hibernating in the outreaches of Nova Scotia), then it will be harder to translate the successes you get from the course back into your day-to-day life. My experience is there is no real difference between those who take these types of extra precautions (unless necessary) and those who do not, at least in terms of success, but people who do take lots of extra precautions tend to get a little more anxious about how to integrate their success back into their daily lives once they have completed the course.

Prescription Medication

The next piece of pre-planning looks at prescription medication use for sleep. If you are taking sleeping tablets or some other medication to help you sleep, should you come off them before or after the course, if at all? That decision is yours to make and I would suggest with some lengthy discussion with your GP or PCP. What I would say is that you should make that decision, either way, and stick with it throughout the course.

We know that changing too many behaviours in one go decreases the likelihood of us being able to manage any one of those changes well and so it is best if you pre-plan whether you will stay on the medication, or not, before you start the course. What I do tend to find is that, by the time someone has got to see me, they usually want to give up their sleep medications, if they are on them, as they feel that either they do not work for them anymore or they don't like taking sleep medications and want an alternative non-pharmacological solution. If you do decide that you want to come off your sleep medication, you MUST do this in consultation with your GP or PCP. They will be able to help you by advising how much to reduce the dosage and over what period of time to do this. How long should you be off the sleep medications before you start the course? I would say at least two weeks, so that when you complete your Pre-course Sleep Diary, it will be a better reflection of how you are sleeping now, without the medication.

What if you decide to stay on the medication? It is fine; my main consideration at this point is the same issue that I highlighted earlier – it may be a little more difficult to integrate or translate those successes back into your life, following completion of the course, without the medication.

The other thing I will say about sleep medication is we can sometimes get into a bit of a Catch-22 when we take it, especially over a long time. What I mean by that is, in my experience, a small number of people will say that they would prefer to stay on their sleep medication throughout treatment and this generally occurs for one of two main reasons: either the individual says that it does afford some relief in terms of sleep 'every now and then' or the individual has tried coming off the sleep medication in the past but the insomnia came right back.

Let's look at these two issues in a little more depth. In terms of the first statement, remember what I said about night-to-night variability in people with insomnia, as well as in good sleepers (page 37)? So, what we may be seeing here is the 'odd' but predictable reasonable night of sleep due to 'normal' variations in sleep patterns and it may not actually be due to the sleep medication working. Think about it this way: remember when I talked about the sleep homeostat and that it builds and builds (increasing sleep pressure) and only resets itself when we have slept (see page 14)? Eventually the sleep pressure will get to such a high point that the individual will sleep irrespective of whether they have insomnia or not. The individual may be attributing that night of reasonable sleep to the medication unnecessarily.

As for the second statement, the thing to bear in mind here is that the insomnia you may experience (not everyone does) when you come off your sleep medications is not the same insomnia that you had previously 'coming back'. This new period of insomnia is quite specific and is what we call 'rebound insomnia' in that it is the actual withdrawal from the sleep medication that precipitates this period of sleep disturbance, either chemically or through anxiety, and not a relapse per se. In most cases this should resolve itself before the two-week threshold of a sleep disturbance is up.

What Kind of Sleeper Do You Want to Be?

As you may have noticed, from my perspective, the pre-planning stage largely revolves around what kind of sleeper you want to be on completion of the course. What we are aiming for here is a situation where you are sleeping better and no longer worried, angry or miserable when thinking about bed or when getting into bed, or indeed, when you are going to sleep. Where the course itself will help you manage all of those worries and concerns (as well as the sleep itself), the more precautions you take (unless absolutely necessary as in the occupations I have talked about above), the more fragile you will believe the success of the course has been for you. That is not ideal to me, as seeing your success as 'fragile' will only increase the chances that you are likely to have a relapse in the future through anxiety.

The question of what kind of sleeper you want to be also comes up a great deal when we talk about partners and whether or not to stay in a separate bedroom during the course. It is quite common, when practical and possible, for people with insomnia to sleep apart from their partners for various reasons, with the main issue being that the person with insomnia does not want to disturb their partner during the night by tossing and turning, turning the lights on to read or watch TV in bed, etc. If you are not already sleeping separately and, assuming you have a partner of course, when you read the instructions on Day 1 and Day 2 of the course I can tell you that you will be even more tempted to go to sleep in another room, if at all possible. Before you do this, my question remains the same, what kind of sleeper do you want to be on completion of the course? If your goal is to get back into the same bedroom as your partner, if you have been sleeping apart, or indeed if you have never left the bedroom and want to continue to be in the same bedroom in the future, then you should really complete the course in the same bed. This, naturally, is a discussion you will want to have with your partner as preparing them can be just as, if not more, integral to success.

What You Will Need for the Course

The final thing we need to talk about in terms of your pre-planning is a little more practical. These are the actual physical things that you will need to complete the course. The first thing is a calculator. The course requires quite a few calculations in order to both determine your personal sleep plan, any adaptations or modifications needed to the plan and for working out the odds of something occurring when we look at catastrophic thinking at night (see page 143). In each case a simple calculator will be sufficient but invaluable. I will provide, where necessary, examples of how to do the calculations, in addition to showing you the equations themselves. The other things you will need are a pen, to complete your diaries (both Sleep and Cognitive Control Diaries) and a notepad. I always find a new notepad, dedicated solely to the course, is the best bet as you can keep any notes, calculations, written activities and Cognitive Control Diaries together in one place.

Preparing Others

Going back to partners for the moment, although there is only a small amount of evidence, what does exist suggests that partners can influence the success of courses like this one quite a bit. From providing physical support – such as buying fruit teas to replace coffee, as was the case for one individual – to emotional support – such as the partner telling the person with insomnia that they could see the benefits of the course in terms of improved mood, as in the case of another individual – even small things can make a really big impact.

From a study I conducted a couple of years ago (alongside Dr Vincent Deary and Dr Wendy Troxel), I have provided a list below of the top 10 most common forms of positive, and negative, support that have been shown to influence the outcome of a full six-week programme of CBT-I which are just as applicable here.

	Positive Support		Negative Support
1	Woke me if I was having a nap	1	Expressed concerns that treatment may only be temporary
2	Dissuaded me from quitting	2	Does not believe in CBT-I
3	Stopped me from using technology in the bedroom	3	Complained about me leaving the bedroom during the night
4	Believed in my ability to cope with CBT-I	4	Allowed me to sleep in occasionally
5	Motivated me to keep going	5	Insisted bedtime routines should stay the same
6	Helped me to find things to do at night	6	Said I was hard to live with because I was so tired
7	Understands why sleep hygiene is so important	7	Voiced concerns that I was not getting better
8	Stayed up later with me at night	8	Said I should stay in bed and try to sleep
9	Made positive comments about my improved mood	9	Will not see someone about their snoring
10	Asked about the content of sessions	10	Would not keep me company at night

As you can see, the biggest barriers from partners, reported by patients, centred on resistance to, or concern over, the impact that changes to routine, environment or behaviour could have on their existing relationship. In these situations, this could be easily managed by providing information for partners about CBT-I and, specifically, the reasons why it is important for you to change some of your existing routines, habits and behaviours. I would suggest that you ask your partner to read a few sections of the book so they can get an idea of why we will be asking you to make those changes. Specifically, I would recommend What Is Insomnia? (page 32), How Insomnia Develops (page 45) and What Does Insomnia Actually Look Like? (page 51), to start with.

Following that, it would be really helpful for you both to explore your partner's expectations, as well as your own and, where necessary and practical, address any concerns about the content of the course before you begin. One way to do this would be to compile a list, like the one above, outlining what help you feel would be beneficial and what may not be helpful to you, and then get your partner to do the same.

Start at the top and work down through each suggestion or comment, identify the potential issue and see if there is a resolution that you are both comfortable with. You may have noticed that I did not use the word 'compromise' but 'resolution' instead. This was deliberate, as you should not compromise on the things that I will be asking you to do, otherwise the course is not going to work as well, if at all, for you.

Here, I am asking you both to identify potential barriers and challenges and find ways forward that do not result in a watered-down version of this course. A good example of how this can be achieved came up quite recently for me. In this case, the husband, Max was really uncomfortable about going to bed on his own but also felt that he could not wait up until it was time for his wife, Juliana to go to bed, according to her personal sleep plan, because he had to be up very early for work. He also felt that going to bed alone, albeit for a short amount of time, could damage their relationship as they had always gone to bed together at the same time for the last seven years. I came to the conclusion whereby they would use my version of 'cuddle time' (see page 18). At what was their previous 'normal' bedtime, they would both get into bed but with two caveats; there would be no intention or effort by Juliana to sleep at this time and, after 15 or so minutes, she would leave the bedroom. The problem was resolved without damaging the course or their relationship and they both did really well.

Of course, partners are not the only arena where you can get additional support while doing the course. The decision to tell people around you that you are doing the course is yours to make, but friends, family and co-workers can all be great additional sources of help and inspiration.

My final word on this issue of support is 'alliance over reliance'. The study I mentioned above also showed that some partners can become overly invested in their partner's treatment and this could also negatively affect the outcome of treatment.

A good example of this was highlighted in one interview with a patient (Simon) in which he said that his partner took 'full' responsibility for making sure he did not fall asleep on the sofa in the early evening, which he was prone to doing. On several occasions he did indeed fall asleep on the sofa but his partner did not wake him, believing that even a small amount of sleep was beneficial for him. I recall the phrase Simon's partner Steve used was 'at least he is getting some sleep, that's good, right?' This is not the case, as falling asleep on the sofa would have the same effect on this patient's sleep as having a nap late in the day (see page 14).

In another case, the partner (Dominic) would ask his girlfriend (Amrita) every night, just as they got into bed, how she was feeling about her insomnia and asked her, every morning, as soon as she woke, how she had slept the previous night. This was not only frustrating to Amrita but also made her think about her insomnia all day resulting in increasing amounts of sleep preoccupation.

I do believe there is a balance that needs to be struck between someone being supportive but not overly intrusive and certainly not 'taking responsibility' for the other person's treatment, and someone being resistant or even obstructive to their partner's treatment. It's about discussing those issues and resolving them before you start the course.

Sleep Hygiene

You may have heard of, read about or even incorporated sleep hygiene into your life already. In fact, more and more, when I see individuals with insomnia they will tell me, usually at the first meeting, that they have tried sleep hygiene and it did not work. The first thing to say about sleep hygiene, and what I say to patients who tell me they have tried it already with no success, is that they are right. It is very unlikely that poor sleep hygiene caused your insomnia and also unlikely that following all the principles of good sleep hygiene will, on their own, fix your insomnia. Think about it this way, there are a significant number of people out there who do not practise good sleep hygiene; in fact they do the complete opposite to what we recommend, and they sleep just fine.

So, you may ask, why are we bothering to talk about it at all? The reason is that, although sleep hygiene will not fix your insomnia, when you have completed all the techniques that follow in Part 2, over the next week, you are likely to see better results if you practise good sleep hygiene. Moreover, having good sleep hygiene may offer a certain level of 'good sleep' in the future. What do we mean by sleep hygiene? This is a series of guidelines that help promote a sleep-healthy environment (the bedroom) and routine.

The Bedroom

The bedroom should be kept cool, dark and quiet – we know that heat, light and noise can all wake an individual up but, more importantly, these three things don't necessarily have to wake us up in order to disrupt our sleep (as I outlined in Cortical Arousal on page 58). We know that heat, light and noise can fragment our sleep and not allow us to consolidate the deep refreshing sleep that we need.

Cool, Dark and Quiet

It is one thing to say cool, dark and quiet, but in some circumstances this is going to be tricky and we may need to think creatively. We may not want, or afford, to have expensive blackout blinds or curtains, so perhaps a good eyemask will do the job instead. Similarly, there may be circumstances where complete darkness is not ideal, so having some form of low but visible lighting – for example, to prevent trips and falls during the night – in a hallway may be helpful.

Similarly, where it may not be practical to keep windows open at night, perhaps keeping them open a couple of hours before bedtime, with the curtains closed, will help maintain a cool environment, especially in the summer months. Also, it is likely that you will not be able to reduce the noise outside the bedroom (for example, traffic or a tree where the birds sing from early in the morning) so good earplugs may be a really helpful way forward.

One great item that can help with both noise and heat is an electric fan. The fan not only cools, but also provides a certain level of background white noise and we know that white noise is helpful for masking a noisy environment when you have no opportunity to reduce noise or when earplugs may not be a practical solution (for example, as in the case of caregivers).

What I would say here is that some people cannot tolerate any form of noise in the bedroom, even white noise. This is an issue, in my view, of heightened cortical arousal. So would a fan be a good idea in these circumstances? My answer is still yes but we need to 'normalise' that sound for you. The way we can do this is through a process of desensitisation. So, record the noise from the fan, about 20–30 minutes' worth, and then play it back to yourself as many times as you like during the day over the next week or so, when you are feeling most awake and alert. This process, given enough playbacks, will normalise the sound and then the fan, or if you want to buy a white-noise machine instead, should no longer be a problem.

Bedding and Mattresses

I get asked quite a lot about mattresses, duvets or comforters, pillows and sheets, what the best types of mattress are and what the best material fibres for bedding are to help you sleep. The answer is a simple one: whichever works best for you. It's a funny thing, but we don't tend to spend a lot of time choosing a mattress or our bedding, even though we probably spend more time in our beds than in our cars – and you would not normally buy a car in under an hour.

In terms of mattresses, my advice is to go to a store and try out as many as it takes before you find one that works for you. Remember to evaluate the mattress when you are on your side(s) as well as on your back as we do tend to shift position a fair amount during the night. Oh, and if you have a significant other, don't be shy; get them to try the mattress with you at the same time.

Duvets/comforters are another area where most of us don't tend to spend a great deal of time doing background research. I am not going to get into a discussion on natural fibres versus synthetic fibres, as both types have advantages and disadvantages, but what I would say is think about temperature changes over the year. Personally, I like the double-layer duvets as both together serve me really well in winter and I can remove one for the summer months. Additionally, if you get too cold or hot at night it is a lot easier, and certainly less disruptive to your sleep, to throw the duvet off or add another layer on than it is to get out of bed to turn the heating up or down or to open or close a window.

The final thing I will say about duvets, especially if you have a significant other, is it may be worth investing in two and getting each one a size larger than the space it occupies. For example, our bed is a king size and so we have two king-size duvets on it. Why? Again, for me it is a temperature issue. If I get cold I tend to steal as much of the duvet as possible, cocooning myself and leaving my significant other out in the cold. Then, about an hour or so later, I get too hot and throw the duvet over my side of the bed (out of their reach) so I can retrieve it easily if I get cold again. Unfair, I know, and so a way to address that issue, and any associated grief the next morning, is to each have your own duvet. The reason to have a size larger than the space it occupies, in my opinion, is that it is more likely that, if you get cold in the night, it feels like you have less overall surface area to cover you up if you have access to only one duvet that is half the size of the bed. However, while I do believe the sum is greater than the parts, at least in the case of duvets, I just get bigger parts to offset my own hogging behaviour.

As for pillows, again it is a matter of personal preference as to what type and how many there should be on the bed (I prefer two myself), but it is important to know when your pillow needs replacing. For some reason, not replacing pillows seems to be an issue for men more than for women, and I have been just as guilty of doing this in the past. Men tend to keep the same pillows they have had since they were at school or college and hardly ever replace a pillow. Anyway, to test when it is time to replace a pillow, hold it out in front of you length-ways. If the pillow bends in half, it is dead and it is time for a replacement. In terms of materials, cotton is great as it allows air circulation and is lightweight whereas silk helps regulate your body temperature by cooling you when you are warm and warming you when you are cold. Again, investing in good bedding will not fix your insomnia but it may help a little.

Clocks

The next thing is clock faces, which should not be visible in the bedroom at all. Now, that is not to say that all clocks must be taken out of the bedroom entirely (you can have them turned away or face down), as having an alarm clock in the bedroom can sometimes be a necessity but it appears, by design, that in the modern age humans like to know what time it is, even in the middle of the night.

The problem comes when we wake in the night; we will check the time and then calculate how much time we have left before we have to get up. Frequently this leads to worry and concern and a tendency to 'clockwatch' for the rest of the night (for example, it is 4am I have 3 hours' sleep left, it is 4.30am I have 2½ hours' sleep left, it is 5am I have 2 hours and so on ...). This is certainly not going to help with getting back off to sleep. My friend and colleague – Dr Michael Perlis was on a flight a couple of years ago and was flipping through the magazine that sells things that you never thought you needed when he saw what was, to me personally, the worst product imaginable for people with insomnia to have in the bedroom. This product, I think it was an alarm clock of sorts, had the capacity to project an enormous clock face on to the bedroom ceiling. Why would you do that to yourself if already you cannot sleep?

Electronics

The traditional wisdom suggests taking all electronics out of the bedroom. There has been a lot of discussion recently about the impact of electronics, in the bedroom and just before bed, on a person's sleep. Specifically, the discussion has focused on how the blue light emitted from our electronics (for example, laptop, phone, tablet) can signal the brain that it is time to be awake and stop the production of melatonin, leading to a delayed sleep onset. In other words, delaying the sleep/wake circadian rhythm.

While I agree, for the most part, I would like to take this issue one step further. The reason I don't like electronics that emit large amounts of blue light being used before bed and specifically in the bedroom is because, in addition to the physiological stimulation caused by the blue light, there is likely to be psychological stimulation as well, which can be just as disruptive, if not even more so, in my experience. Checking email, using social media, writing reports, etc. are activities that are likely to get your brain thinking at a time when it should be winding down for sleep. Moreover, with these forms of communication, particularly email and social media, there appears to be that immediacy where we are either expected to respond almost immediately to something or are waiting for an immediate response from someone else. I have seen, first hand, how disruptive that can be to sleep, and this appears to be an increasing problem for younger adults.

In fact, I tend to advise setting yourself a regular cut-off time, around 1½–2 hours before bedtime, when you should stop using all those electronics (except the television which you can use as long as it is not in the bedroom) irrespective of whether you wear blue-light blockers or have screens on your electronics that filter out blue light. If you also inform friends and family that is what you are doing, that should also reduce their stress and anxiety about getting an immediate response, unless necessary. Now, what I have said here is about using electronics before bed and in bed. I have absolutely no problem with electronics being in the bedroom, as in some circumstances it could be even more stressful to have them elsewhere (such as in case of emergencies or if the children are out). Just keeping them out of useable reach I have found can be sufficient alternative.

Pets

The final issue we need to discuss in relation to the sleep environment is pets. Don't get me wrong, I love pets (our cat

Harry, or little man, as he is otherwise known, is a huge part of my world) but having a pet in the bedroom, let alone on, or dare I say, in, the bed can be very disruptive to your sleep. Most pets are either nocturnal or have very different sleep/wake patterns to us humans. As such, your pets are likely to be up and about jumping on and off the bed while you are sleeping and in many cases this can wake us up or can fragment our sleep. If you do have pets in the bedroom, consider setting up an alternative space, outside the bedroom, for your pet to sleep in and train them to sleep there. If that is not a possibility, for whatever reason, then training your pet to sleep in the bedroom but not on the bed is an acceptable, although not ideal, alternative.

The Routine

Here we talk about some of the things you eat, drink and do that can increase the chances that you will either have difficulties getting off to sleep or wake up more frequently during the night. The first three are caffeine, nicotine and alcohol.

Caffeine is a drug that works by reducing our levels of tiredness. This appears to be a great solution if you are sleepy in the daytime but, because caffeine can stay in your system and affect you for quite some time after you have taken it, your natural cues to sleep may be reduced or lost. As such, drinking caffeine, or indeed eating things that contain a lot of caffeine from the afternoon onwards has the potential to negatively impact on your sleep so I tend to ask people to avoid caffeine about eight hours before bedtime.

Similar to caffeine, nicotine is a stimulant and so smoking close to bedtime can also interfere with your body's natural ability to prepare you for sleep. Additionally, if you are awake in the night, nicotine is likely to increase your wakefulness so if you can avoid it you are more likely to get back off to sleep easier.

Alcohol, on the other hand, is a sedative, which certainly sounds appealing if you are having difficulties getting off to sleep. It is worth noting that a lot of people with insomnia try using alcohol to sleep, with disastrous consequences. The problem is the effects of alcohol wear off quite quickly and this leads to increased amounts of light unrefreshing sleep in the second half of the night. Additionally, as alcohol is a diuretic, you are more likely to become dehydrated which increases sleep fragmentation during the second half of the night. So, avoid drinking lots of alcohol close to bedtime and certainly avoid using alcohol as a sleep aid.

Exercise

Exercise is great for sleep and we know from over 40 studies that regular exercise is associated with longer and deeper sleep, even in people who normally sleep well. Similarly, for people with insomnia the studies show that moderate-intensity exercise in the afternoon or early evening is associated with getting off to sleep quicker and increased overall amounts of sleep. The one issue with exercise that we have to bear in mind is doing it too close to bedtime. If you exercise too close to bedtime, I usually say within 2 hours of bedtime, it can sometimes interfere with the sleep process. Remember exercise is one of the three factors that can offset the sleep/wake circadian rhythm and if you exercise too close to bedtime it can delay sleep onset a little.

For some people exercise may be a problem. There may be practical issues (nowhere nearby to exercise, safety) or physical limitations (mobility problems) that can prevent you from exercising later in the afternoon or early evening. In those instances a hot (not scalding) bath, about 2 hours before bedtime, can be a beneficial alternative in terms of sleep, but unfortunately not in terms of fitness. The reason a hot bath (but not a shower) helps with sleep is that it warms up the body quite quickly but, and just as it is in the case of exercise, following that temperature peak your body temperature reduces quite rapidly and this mimics the body temperature changes that occur naturally with the opening of the sleep gate. So it's almost as if you were tricking your physical body into feeling extra ready for sleep. This rapid reduction in body temperature (I call it a temperature cascade) occurs around 2 hours after the bath or, in the case of exercise, approximately 2 hours after you have finished exercising.

Diet

As with exercise, eating a heavy meal close to bedtime is not going to help with getting off to sleep as your body will be trying to achieve two opposing biological processes at the same time – in this case, digestion and sleep. I usually say try not to eat a heavy meal within 2 hours of bedtime. That said, it is equally important not to go to bed hungry as that can also wake you up. A night-time snack is fine and incorporating cereals, nuts, soft fruits and/or bananas (the greener the better because, as it ripens, the banana loses its capacity to stimulate the production of melatonin) can actually help you sleep as they can increase the levels of melatonin in the body.

Finally, we should look at liquid intake. Although it is not a good idea to go to bed thirsty, to avoid the need to go to the bathroom in the night it may be a good idea to reduce your liquid intake from the early evening onwards. Having to get up in the night to use the bathroom is a specific problem, that we call Nocturia, that starts to occur more frequently as we get older, and specifically for men, which can be very disruptive to your sleep.

The Pre-course Sleep Diary

Okay, so now can we get going? The answer is yes and we are going to start with how to record your sleep throughout the course. The Sleep Diary (both Pre-course and On-course) is probably the most important tool you will need in order to do this course. In fact, I feel so strongly that the Sleep Diary is so integral to success that, when I am doing therapy (either in practice or in research), I will start each session by asking to see the Sleep Diary and if there is no diary, there is no therapy that day and I am not alone in that philosophy.

It will seem like a pain at first but you have to stick with it as it will be invaluable in helping you identify any patterns in your sleep that may otherwise have gone unnoticed, how your insomnia is manifesting, your specific sleep schedule over this course, and, importantly, over time it will be an excellent marker of your progress.

More and more I am being asked whether 'sleep trackers' (the products usually worn on the wrist that use technology based upon movements, like actigraphy, to make assumptions about our sleep) can be used instead of Sleep Diaries. My answer at this time is no, unless there are practical limitations to completing the Sleep Diary by hand. Most of the trackers on the market have not yet been tested against the technology that we use (actigraphy or polysomnography). Probably more importantly, what we need here are your impressions of your sleep pattern. As we saw earlier, the diagnosis of insomnia is largely based upon your impressions of your problems sleeping and how your sleep is affecting you in the daytime. For example, we know from actigraphy and polysomnography studies that even 'normal' sleepers wake up a few times in the night, each night, but they will just go back to sleep and don't remember being awake. I can only imagine that, by giving a 'normal' sleeper the news that they were awake that many times in the night, I am going to be creating a lot more people with anxieties around their sleep. In essence, as the technology that exists out there has not been used on people who have insomnia in a systematic way, from my perspective the Sleep Diary remains, for now, the most essential tool to complete the course.

My Sleep Diary - Pre-Course

	Day 1	Day 2	Day 3	Day 4	Day 5	Day 6	Day 7	Ave.
About yesterday								
1) Did you have a nap today (yes / no)?								
1a) If you had a nap what time did you last nap?								
1b) How long did you nap today in total (minutes)?								
2) Did you unintentionally fall asleep at any point today (yes / no)?								
About last night								
3) What time did you intend to go to bed?								
4) What time did you get into bed?								
5) What time did you turn out the lights intending of going to sleep?								
6) How long (minutes) did it take you to fall asleep?								
7) Did you wake in the night (yes / no)?								
7a) If you woke during the night how many times did you wake?								
7b) How long were you awake during the night in total (minutes)?								
About this morning								
8) What time did you wake up (your final awakening)?								
9) How long was this from when you had intended to wake up (minutes)?								
10) What time did you get out of bed?								
11) How would you rate the quality of your sleep last night? (1 = very poor - 5 = excellent)								
12) How refreshed do you feel this morning? (1 = not at all - 5 = extremely refreshed)								
Overall								
Time in Bed								
Total Duration of Time Awake In Bed								
Total Sleep Time								
Sleep Efficiency %								
Number of Awakenings								
Sleep Latency								
Wake After Sleep Onset								

When Should You Complete Your Sleep Diary?

You should complete it every morning, ideally after you have been awake for at least 20 minutes. The reason I say then, and not earlier, is because of a phenomenon called 'sleep inertia'. We have all experienced that period of time, usually lasting up to about 20 minutes from waking, where we feel 'not quite with it'. We are slightly dazed and sluggish and it takes us a little time to get our thoughts together, almost as if we were half asleep and half awake. This, like the hypnic jerk I described on page 20, is quite normal and natural and is just a sign of a less-than-smooth transition from sleep to wakefulness. As such, it is never a good idea to evaluate your sleep during that period as you are going to be less accurate in your estimations and more likely to attribute the inertia, at that moment, to a poor night of sleep. This is especially important if you have insomnia.

If you forget to complete your entry outside, say, a 20–40-minute waking zone, please don't fill it in retrospectively. Leave the whole day blank and monitor for an additional day to compensate. It is important that we have data that is averaged over a significant period of time so that we can account for variability from night to night (as I mentioned earlier, even people with insomnia have the odd good night) as well as an abnormally good or bad sleep period (which we all have from time to time).

The other thing to mention here is about clockwatching. As you will have seen in Sleep Hygiene on page 86, I am going to ask you to make sure there are no visible clocks in your bedroom. So, you may be asking, how can I ask you to complete a Sleep Diary with any degree of accuracy without a clock? Well, where this should not be too much of a problem when recording the times of getting into and out of bed, what about recording times awake during the night? The answer is we really only need your estimate as a starting point from which you can determine how well you are doing later on.

Using the Pre-course Sleep Diary

The Pre-course Sleep Diary is split into three main question sections (yesterday, last night and this morning) and then a fourth section (overall) for all your calculations, which I will come on to.

In the first section, we are mainly asking about napping behaviour. As you saw on page 14, naps that are long (I would say over 30 minutes) or taken late in the day (after lunchtime) can be detrimental to your sleep at night, by sating the sleep homeostat too early, and so this is where you will be able to determine whether the naps you are having, if indeed you are napping, are affecting your sleep. In many cases, when you compare days with naps against days without naps, you will see an association between long late-afternoon naps and problems getting off to sleep at night.

Question 2 asks about unintentional daytime sleeping. If you answered yes to this question, it is essential to get this investigated further by a GP/PCP or other healthcare professional BEFORE you start the course, or indeed, if this occurs at any point during the course you should STOP the course and get this investigated. It is unusual for people with insomnia to unintentionally fall asleep during the daytime. The reason we say that is people with insomnia tend to be 'tired but wired'; in other words, they are generally tired but unable to sleep when given the opportunity. Conversely, people who unintentionally fall asleep or need to sleep during the day tend to be sleepy which is predominantly associated with the DOES category of sleep disorders (see page 64).

The second and third sections of the Pre-course Sleep Diary provide a picture of the sleep you obtained last night and are the basis for calculating how efficient your sleep is (which I will discuss in a moment), while also giving you a sense of your sleep quality and its capacity to rejuvenate you.

Questions 3–6 ask about your usual sleep onset habits. Here it is worth looking at how much time there is between intending to go to bed (Question 3) and the actual time you got into bed (Question 4). The longer the gap between the intention to go to bed and actually getting into bed may be influencing how long it is taking you to get off to sleep (Question 6), especially if what you are doing during that time is physically, psychologically or emotionally stimulating or arousing. You should ask yourself what is preventing you from going to bed when you intended to. If it is a case of not being tired, then that is fine but if it is this something else, can that activity or event be changed or moved to earlier in the day or evening?

The same issue may arise when you examine your intended time to wake up (Question 9) against the actual time you woke up in the morning (Question 8). If you intended to wake up at a certain time but woke up later, perhaps an alarm may be helpful.

Calculating Your Sleep Variables

You will be using the final section of the Pre-course Sleep Diary to provide a quantitative overview of your sleep. Here a calculator is most helpful. I would prefer that you also complete this section every morning, when you complete the other parts of your Sleep Diary but this section can always be completed later if you run out of time in the morning.

The first variable we need is Time in Bed (TIB) and this should be calculated as the amount of time, in minutes, between getting into bed and getting out of bed. In other words, the amount of time that has elapsed between Question 4 (what time I got into bed) and Question 10 (what time I got out of bed). For example, if I got into bed at 11pm and got out of bed at 6am then my time in bed would be 7 hours or 420 minutes.

The next variable is very important as it provides an overview of how much time you are spending at night awake in bed (this is referred to as Time Awake in Bed – TAIB). This will be the summation of (1) the amount of time you were in bed before you fell asleep (the amount of time, in minutes, that has elapsed between getting into bed – Question 4 – and putting the lights out intending to go to sleep – Question 5, plus the amount of time it took you to get off to sleep – Question 6), (2) how long you were awake during the night (Question 7b) and how long you were in bed after you had woken in the morning before you got out of the bed (the difference in minutes between Question 8 and Question 10).

So, let's say that I got into bed at 10pm and I fell asleep 40 minutes later. Then I was awake for 20 minutes in the night. Finally, I woke up at 6am but stayed in bed till 7am. At this point it does not matter what I was doing at any of those times, just how much time I am spending in bed at night awake. So, 40 minutes + 20 minutes + 60 minutes gives me a total TAIB of 120 minutes.

Next is Total Sleep Time (TST). TST is calculated as the amount of time (in minutes) you spent in bed (TIB) minus the amount of time awake, in bed, at night (TAIB). Remember for TAIB it does not matter what you were doing when you were awake, just that you were awake in bed. So, if I am in bed for 420 minutes but I read in bed for 10 minutes, it took me 10 minutes to get off to sleep, I was awake for 10 minutes in the night and then I spent 30 minutes in the morning in bed trying to get back to sleep after waking up, then my TST will be my TIB (420 minutes) – (10 + 10 + 10 + 30) = 360 minutes.

The next variable you need is Sleep Efficiency (SE). This tells you how efficiently you are sleeping. The equation for SE is as follows: TST/TIB x 100.

I know this is a pain but please bear with it. So, going back to the last example, if my TST is 360 minutes and my TIB is 420 minutes, then 360/420 x 100 = 85.71%. This shows that I am 85.71% sleep efficient, which actually is not bad at all.

It is very important to be able to calculate your own Sleep Efficiency as this is the key calculation you will be using throughout the entire course to tailor your specific sleep plan and so I would recommend practising this equation a few times. I have also included an example of a completed Sleep Diary on page 109 which you can also use to practise with.

The final variables relate to your symptoms. These are: Number of Awakenings – how many times did you wake up in the night? This is quite self-explanatory and can be taken directly from Question 7a (how many times I woke in the night). The next is called Sleep Latency (SL) – how long were you awake in bed before falling asleep after turning out the lights? This is the difference in minutes between getting into bed and falling asleep (the answer to Question 6) and Wake After Sleep Onset (WASO) – how much time I was awake during the night (the answer to Question 7b plus the difference, in minutes, between Questions 8 and 10).

Some Common Questions Answered

Do I Have to Do the Whole Course?

The main question I usually get is, 'Do I have to do the whole course?' As for this question, I emphatically say yes, if indeed you are a candidate for the full course. My rationale for this is that, if you start with the first technique, you are likely to see some improvement in your sleep and there may well be a temptation to stop there and not realise the full potential benefits of the course. That, to me, would be a wasted opportunity. To me, this course is like taking a course of antibiotics in the sense that you should complete the whole course even though you may be tempted to stop when you see some benefits early on.

Is the Order of the Techniques Important?

So, why have I chosen the order that I have and is it important to follow it in the order which I have presented it? In answer to these questions, the reason for my ordering is simple; I have chosen what I believe are the most powerful techniques first (sleep rescheduling and stimulus control), then the next most powerful (cognitive control) and so forth through the week. I have specifically chosen sleep rescheduling as Day 1 as, in my view, it requires the most time to personalise and get to grips with, whereas stimulus control and the other cognitive techniques need a little more planning but less personalising. So, yes, this order is important and should be followed, unless indicated otherwise.

Can I Go at My Own Pace?

The next question I usually get asked when I outline the course is, 'Do I have to adopt a new technique every day or can I go at my own pace?' The simple answer is you can go at your own pace if that is what you want to do. That said, please remember that, as the course is additive (you don't stop using a technique after you have learnt it, you just add the new technique on top), you should continue doing all the prior techniques during the time in between in addition to completing your Sleep Diary every day. For example, if you wanted to leave a week between the techniques outlined on Day 2 – Stimulus Control and Day 3 – Cognitive Control, you would continue doing all the activities from Day 1 – Sleep Rescheduling and the stimulus control techniques from Day 2 and then incorporate the cognitive control technique from Day 3 when you are ready to continue. What I would say is that if you do decide to leave time between sessions, read the titration rules on Day 6 and titrate your sleep rescheduling routine at the end of each week (see page 151) irrespective of what stage you are at.

When Should I Read and Implement Each Technique?

The final thing I get asked and that we need to discuss at this point is when, each day, should you read and implement the relevant technique.

Well, I would say that I would very rarely see someone with insomnia, for CBT-I, after 7pm (even when I am doing it as part of my research) and there are two reasons for this. Firstly, I usually want to go home by then but secondly, and more importantly, I usually want the individual to implement the techniques and strategies that we have discussed on that same day. As such, doing a session late in the evening means that it may be difficult for the person to digest what we have discussed, practise and then integrate the technique that same day. So, what I would say is give yourself enough time to read through the section, at least once, so reading the relevant section by the early evening would be best.

A Note for Individuals with Paradoxical Insomnia

If it is the case that you have Paradoxical Insomnia, have seen a BSM and had the go-ahead for the course it is NOT recommended that you do the Day 1 activities (sleep rescheduling) but instead replace that with the section on managing sleep distortions INSTEAD (see page 115) and then complete the rest of the course as normal. Additionally, people with Paradoxical Insomnia do not need to do the sleep titration activity on Day 6 as that is tied to sleep rescheduling. However, they SHOULD DO the progressive muscle relaxation exercise on Day 6 (see page 154).

The Course

Day 1 Sleep Rescheduling

Okay, let's start. You may have heard of something called Sleep Restriction Therapy and in essence that is what we are going to be doing here. So, why have I chosen a different name?

The reason I have done this is because I do not believe that Sleep Restriction Therapy is an appropriate term, as that is NOT what we are doing here. Even the originator of this aspect of the course, Professor Art Spielman, termed it 'Restriction of Time in Bed'. On page 50 I talked about how excessive time in bed is bad for sleep and perpetuates insomnia and that is what we are going to address here.

On page 50 I used Donn's analogy of stretching dough to exemplify the point about the influence of going to bed early and having a lie-in on sleep, so let's continue from there. At the moment (from where we left off the description), the dough is representing your sleep as it looks now (very light sleep with lots of time awake and large vulnerable points to awakening) as a result of stretching out your time in bed. If you want to thicken the dough in order to make it more consolidated and get rid of the holes and vulnerability points, what should you do? Let's first put forward the caveat that we cannot increase the amount of dough we have, as that is our biological sleep need, which cannot be changed. So, what we have to do is squish the dough back together to make it thicker, as it was before we stretched it.

Just as we are not adding extra dough, we are not taking away any of the dough either so we are not actually restricting your sleep, just the amount of time you spend in bed. The difficulty we have is that I just don't know how much to squish it back by in order to get you to 'normal' sleep, as I do not know what the dough looked like before you had insomnia and this is where together we have to tailor you a personalised sleep plan.

You may now be asking about the mild sleep deprivation that I talked about earlier in relation to sleep rescheduling and where that comes in. Think about it this way: even though we are not restricting your sleep per se, we will be restricting the opportunity for sleep. And so, just like having jet lag, it is going to take a couple of days for your body to adjust to this new routine and you are likely, at least for the first few days, to still have problems with getting off to sleep or waking in the night, albeit to a lesser extent. That is where the mild sleep deprivation comes from. As such, the thing we need to be prepared for is that things are likely to get a little worse before they get better.

The first thing we will need to get going with sleep rescheduling and creating your personal sleep plan is your completed Pre-course Sleep Diary. If you do not have at least one continuous week of your Pre-course Sleep Diary completed, you should NOT start the course and should wait until you have a minimum of one week (preferably two). As I said earlier, no Sleep Diary no treatment (and that also counts for this course, although it will be quite difficult for me to enforce!).

We now need to determine what your average Total Sleep Time (TST) has been over the pre-course period. Remember, TST is calculated as: Time in Bed (TIB) minus time awake, in bed, during the night (TAIB).

The example of a completed Sleep Diary below may help here. As we can see, this individual (Barry) has on Day 1 a TIB of 510 minutes and a TAIB of 100 minutes (0 minutes in bed before lights out, 40 minutes to get off to sleep, 60 minutes awake in the night and 0 minutes in bed awake before he got up). This suggests a Total Sleep Time (TST) on Day 1 of 410 minutes (TIB = 510 − TAIB = 100). For Day 2 we can see Barry has a TIB of 465 minutes and a total TAIB of 100 minutes (15 minutes in bed before lights out, 30 minutes to get off to sleep, 55 minutes awake in the night and 0 minutes in bed awake before he got up) suggesting a TST of 365 minutes.

If we now add all the TSTs from the week together, we get an overall TST of 2,745 minutes and the average over the

Example Sleep Dairy - Pre-Course

	Day 1	Day 2	Day 3	Day 4	Day 5	Day 6	Day 7	Ave.
About yesterday								
1) Did you have a nap today (yes / no)?	No	No	No	No	No	No	No	
1a) If you had a nap what time did you last nap?	N/A	N/A	N/A	N/A	N/A	N/A	N/A	
1b) How long did you nap today in total (minutes)?	N/A	N/A	N/A	N/A	N/A	N/A	N/A	
2) Did you unintentionally fall asleep at any point today (yes / no)?	No	No	No	No	No	No	No	
About last night								
3) What time did you intend to go to bed?	23:00	23:00	23:00	23:00	23:00	23:00	23:00	
4) What time did you get into bed?	22:30	23:15	23:30	22:45	23:00	24:00	24:30	
5) What time did you turn out the lights intending of going to sleep?	22:30	23:30	24:00	23:30	23:30	24:00	01:00	
6) How long (minutes) did it take you to fall asleep?	40	30	5	10	10	0	20	
7) Did you wake in the night (yes / no)?	Yes	Yes	Yes	Yes	Yes	No	Yes	
7a) If you woke during the night how many times did you wake?	2	1	2	1	3	N/A	2	
7b) How long were you awake during the night in total (minutes)?	60	55	50	45	100	0	70	
About this morning								
8) What time did you wake up (your final awakening)?	07:00	07:00	07:00	07:00	07:00	08:30	08:30	
9) How long was this from when you had intended to wake up (minutes)?	0	0	0	0	0	0	30	
10) What time did you get out of bed?	07:00	07:00	07:00	07:00	07:00	09:00	09:30	
11) How would you rate the quality of your sleep last night (1 = very poor - 5 = excellent)	2	2	3	2	2	4	1	
12) How refreshed do you feel this morning (1 = not at all - 5 = extremely refreshed)	1	2	2	2	2	3	2	
Overall								
Time in Bed	510	465	450	495	480	540	540	
Total Duration of Time Awake in Bed	100	100	85	100	140	30	180	
Total Sleep Time	410	365	365	395	340	510	360	392
Sleep Efficiency %	80.39%	78.28%	81.11%	79.80%	70.83%	94.44%	66.67%	78.79
Number of Awakenings	2	1	2	1	3	N/A	2	1.57
Sleep Latency	40	30	5	10	10	0	20	16.4
Wake After Sleep Onset	60	55	50	45	100	0	100	58.6

week (dividing by 7) works out at a TST of 392.14 minutes per night. I am going to round that down to 392 minutes.

So, now you need to work out your average TST. Remember, I said we were not going to restrict your total sleep time, so your average TST will now become your Prescribed Time in Bed (PTIB) in your personalised sleep plan. In the case of Barry, his PTIB is now 392 minutes.

This is probably the MOST important aspect of sleep rescheduling. Irrespective of what your Sleep Diary calculations suggest, from the data averaged over the week(s), you should NEVER EVER restrict your time in bed (PTIB) to fewer than 5 hours (300 minutes) per night.

So, what should you do if your average over the week is fewer than 5 hours? If your average Total Sleep Time, over the pre-assessment period, works out to be fewer than 5 hours (say, 240 minutes or 270 minutes/4 or 4½ hours) you give yourself a full 5 hours (300 minutes) as your Prescribed Time in Bed. Why? Well, we know that sleeping 4 hours, or fewer, a night can have quite a serious impact on your ability to function properly (your memory, attention, problem solving, reaction time when responding to risk, decision-making ability are all negatively affected) the next day and this amount of sleep can also negatively impact on your immune system's ability to function and protect you from illness. So, we have to set a benchmark of 5 hours (300 minutes) to be on the safe side.

Right, so now you should have worked out your PTIB, which of course will be 5 hours, or longer. The next thing we need to do is set your bedtime and wake time according to your PTIB. The important thing to do here is 'anchor' your PTIB to the morning and keep to that time throughout the course. In other words, think about your week and determine the time you have to be awake by every morning. Most people set this as the time when they need to get up and get ready for work, getting the kids ready for school or getting to college/university. If that is not the case, because either you are retired or not working, you still need to set a time that will work for you.

Set that time as your Prescribed Time Out of Bed (PTOB) first and then work backwards to determine your Prescribed Time to Bed (PTTB). Why do we anchor to the morning? Well, as you will see later, when we further personalise your personal sleep plan, we are likely to be allowing additional Time in Bed (TIB) and you may not be able to add this to the morning as you would already have to be up to start your day (for example, to get ready for work). Alongside that, the other reason we anchor to the morning is we know that keeping to a regular wake-up time is more beneficial for keeping the sleep homeostat and sleep/wake circadian rhythm in concert, compared with your bedtime.

So, how I determine an anchor point is by asking the individual the earliest time they have to be out of bed in the morning in a typical week. Going back to our example, let's say Barry has to be up and out of bed by 7am (his PTOB) and his average PTIB, derived from his Pre-course Sleep Diary, is 392 minutes. So, Barry's PTTB is now 12.28am. I am sure Barry is not going to argue with me over 2 minutes, so I would suggest his PTTB is 12.30am, as I usually round up or down to the nearest 5-minute time point (for example, 11.35pm instead of 11.37 or 1.15am instead of 1.12).

At this point you need to determine your personal PTTB and PTOB and then ask yourself whether that is realistically manageable for the next seven days. If not, we may need to look at the anchor time again because it is absolutely vital to keep the PTOB at the same every day, yes, even on non-work days, vacation days, weekends, etc. Remember, we are not going to change or increase the amount of time you are allowed to be in bed (i.e. your PTIB) at this point as that would then give you a watered-down version of sleep rescheduling which is not going to help you; we are just going to tweak the timing of it to make it more manageable for you. Remember also that this is the only point throughout the entire course at which we can tweak the anchor time.

I will be upfront about this. This aspect of the course is the hardest part for both the person with insomnia and usually the therapist, even if delivered face to face, as well. Many of those

I have trained over the years negotiate the amount of PTIB with their patients when they first begin doing full CBT-I, or a briefer version of it, like this one. The reason I know this is because, when I am reviewing their notes and a patient does not appear to be getting any better, this is the first place I look for an answer. Any negotiation of PTIB is ultimately not good for the therapist (they feel like they have failed when the patient does not get better) or for the patient (they want to get better and don't). Let's apply the same principles as any typical encounter with a healthcare professional. If you are told that you need to take a certain medication at a certain dose at a certain time in order to get better, are you going to negotiate the dosage and timing with your GP/PCP? And, if you do manage to negotiate a new timing or dosage, the GP/PCP is likely to advise you that the medication is not going to be as effective, if effective at all. The same principle applies here.

What Happens If I Know That I Am Just Not Going to Be Able to Do This?

You may be saying at this point that this is simply something you cannot do or are not prepared to do. If it is the former, that is okay and this is the case for some people, especially when they feel that, with some extra support, they may be able to do sleep rescheduling. Firstly, I would say please don't give up on CBT-I altogether. In this case I would certainly explore getting individual face-to-face treatment from a Behavioural Sleep Medicine specialist. If it is the latter (not being prepared to do sleep rescheduling), I would say two things: firstly, please don't just ignore sleep rescheduling and continue the course. Without the sleep rescheduling you are not likely to see the full benefits of this course and be disappointed by the end. Secondly, and lastly, maybe consider coming back to the course when you feel that you are prepared to do sleep rescheduling.

What Am I Supposed to Do Until My PTTB?

So, now we should have your prescribed sleep param-
eters (PTTB and PTOB) to fit in with your PTIB. The next
comment I usually get is, 'What the hell am I going to do till x
o'clock?' Here, there are two schools of thought. The first school
suggests that you should do something calming, relaxing and/or
quiet in a dimly lit, comfortable environment. In other words, do
nothing that is physically, psychologically or emotionally arousing. Examples of these kinds of activities include: handwriting
letters, reading, listening to easy music, knitting, etc. The other
school of thought, the one I subscribe to, suggests you can do
anything you like with five main exceptions: no pornography,
work, food, exercise or blue light.

Now I feel that I need to explain myself. Firstly, I have no issues
with pornography but if it is the only time you can indulge in it,
then this is likely to reinforce your insomnia as having a specific
purpose and that is never a good thing in my view. The same thing
applies for catching up on work. As Donn says, 'Never give your
insomnia a purpose.' As for food (as in a meal, not a snack), exercise (as in moderate intensity or vigorous exercise, not walking
from one room to another) and blue light (blue light-emitting
devices close to the face, not the television 10 feet away), as we
saw earlier (page 90), each of these factors can disrupt the sleep/
wake circadian rhythm and I don't want to create a Circadian
Rhythm Disorder to go alongside your insomnia. It should also
go without saying that you should not drink caffeinated drinks or
eat caffeinated snacks, smoke or drink alcohol at this time either.

The other thing NOT to do, whichever school you subscribe
to, is nap. Remember what we said about napping close to
bedtime? If you nap, even a brief nap, during this time it is just
going to add to your difficulty sleeping later on by sating the
sleep homeostat. This is one of the reasons I prefer you to be
doing something enjoyable at this time, as there is, at least to
my mind, less of a chance that you will fall asleep. This does

bring me on to talk about 'the dreaded sofa'. When I have asked people how they got on with their sleep rescheduling, the one thing I do tend to find is that those people who recline on the sofa during this time – you know, like they are waiting for a modelling photo shoot – are the ones that tend to fall asleep and end up not getting the full benefits from sleep rescheduling or indeed stimulus control (which you will read about tomorrow). What I tend to say is, if you are going to use the sofa or a comfy chair, don't recline, sit up straight on the edge of the sofa or chair. That way, if you start to doze off the likelihood is that you will wake yourself up as opposed to falling asleep.

Apart from those things (napping, pornography, a meal, a bout of exercise, excessive blue light or work), you can do almost anything you like as long as it is safe for you to do, does not cause harm to others and is not going to disrupt someone else's sleep. What I usually do is get people to compile a bucket list of all the movies they have always wanted to watch or a television series that they want to catch up on, to watch on a TV (not on a computer, tablet or phone) during this time. The decision as to what you choose to do during this extra time is entirely yours to make, but I would say that I don't want you to feel that this is a punishment, something that has to be endured, but rather an opportunity to do at least interesting things with the extra time you have.

I recall an incident recently when I told a patient (Patrick) that he could do anything during this time, except what I have just outlined to you. The look of relief on his face was so palpable that I had to ask why he looked so relieved. He thought I was going to tell him to sit in a dark corner somewhere reading a magazine or doing something that he felt was 'really dull'. Again, remember when I talked about what kind of sleeper you want to be by the end of the course? Same thing applies here. I am pretty sure some people will disagree with this, but I feel that doing very quiet and non-arousing things before this new bedtime, if that is not who you are, is going to feel a bit like punishment. Moreover, if you do things that are not part of your 'normal', then, to me, that sends the signal that your sleep is fragile, something to be careful around, and I don't think treading on egg shells around your sleep is going to be good for you in the long term. You are still likely to get better if you do things outside your 'norm', agreed, but you are more likely to treat sleep forever more as something vulnerable and fragile, which to me is a recipe for relapse.

The Last Thing You Need to Do on Day 1

The last thing to do today is to calculate your average Sleep Efficiency (SE), Sleep Latency (SL) and Wake After Sleep Onset (WASO) variables from your Pre-course Sleep Diary if you have not already done so this morning. Although these calculations are not needed for implementing sleep rescheduling, they will become increasingly important as we progress, as they will be a good benchmark from which you can track your improvements over the course.

Remember, your average Sleep Efficiency will be the total of TST/TIB x 100 from each day, divided by the number of days completed. It is also important to note that from this point onwards, starting tomorrow morning, we are going to use the On-course Sleep Diary as opposed to the Pre-course Sleep Diary.

Managing Sleep Distortions as an Alternative to Sleep Rescheduling

Here we have an alternative to sleep rescheduling for those individuals who have a case of Paradoxical Insomnia. Remember, if you meet either of the two criteria that I outlined on page 41, you must discuss your insomnia with a Behavioural Sleep Medicine specialist (BSM) before you begin the course. Tell them about this book and the course. A good BSM will understand, determine whether you have Paradoxical

Insomnia, or not, and guide you, hopefully, back to this very part of the book if you do have Paradoxical Insomnia.

What we are going to do here is look at how much of a sleep distortion you have and you are going to examine that yourself over the rest of this week. Time is a funny thing and we can all be both good and bad at estimating time, largely depending upon what we are doing and how much we are focused on what we are doing. The idiom 'time flies when you are having fun' is true – when we do something enjoyable, stimulating or distracting, time appears to pass quite quickly. However, when we are doing something monotonous or when we are waiting for something to happen, the idiom 'a watched pot never boils' seems more appropriate. As I said earlier, it is not the case that a person with Paradoxical Insomnia is mad, or telling lies; it just appears that their ability to perceive sleep as sleep is not as finely tuned as people who do not have Paradoxical Insomnia, in my view, due to increased cortical arousal at night, for whatever reason.

The first thing we need to do is set a regular time for you to go to bed (your Prescribed Time to Bed – PTTB) and get out of bed (your Prescribed Time Out of Bed – PTOB). This should be based upon the average time you have gone to bed and got out of bed during the week(s), from your Pre-course Sleep Diary. This schedule has to be kept for the whole week so be mindful of that before you set those times. It may be best to determine the earliest time you have to be up by when you have commitments the next day (for example, work) and setting that as your PTOB. You will also need to keep a Sleep Diary for this week so I would start using the On-course Sleep Diary from today (detailed in Day 2).

For this technique, I am going to allow you to use your mobile phone, if you have one, in the bedroom, but only as directed. If you do not have a mobile phone or are really uncomfortable about using it in the bedroom after everything I said earlier, a stopwatch or something similar will do just as well. What we need here is something that can record whether you observed an event occurring or not. So, over the next week, when you get into bed at your PTTB, I want you to place the phone on silent, face down, by the bed. You may want to put it under your pillow but I don't really like people doing that for a variety of reasons, one of which being that if it vibrates it may well wake you up unnecessarily.

I would like you to do one of three things, depending upon your main sleep complaint. However, the important thing to do, in each case, is to complete your On-course Sleep Diary the next morning before you look at, or record, the data from your mobile phone or other device.

1. If your main problem is getting off to sleep (initial insomnia), I want you to determine the average amount of time that it took you to get off to sleep that week, from your Pre-course Sleep Diary (the answer to Question 6). Let's say, for argument's sake, that on average it took you 97 minutes to fall asleep that week. Also, record how many nights you went over that average, let's say four times that week. Now, I want you to set an alarm, just a single ping, loud enough to notice if you were awake but not loud enough to wake you up if you were asleep, at 97 minutes, for the whole week. Each morning, after you have completed your On-course Sleep Diary, note down whether you heard the ping, or not. At the end of the week, total the number of nights you heard the ping. Depending on how far off you are from your average (in this case four), this will give you a crude indication of your level of sleep distortion.

2. If your main complaint is lots of awakenings in the night (middle insomnia), then I want you to first calculate from your Pre-course Sleep Diary, on average, from the whole week, how many times you wake up every night (the answer to Question 7a). Let's say that on average you woke up six times every night. So, keep the phone or device by your bed for the next week. Every time you awaken in the night press a dedicated key, just once (please use the hash key or the star key as you do not want to dial a friend, family member or indeed the police in the middle of the night). Each morning, after completing your On-course Sleep

Diary, record how many presses on your phone there were that night. At the end of the week work out how far, on average, you are away from six. That will give you an indication of your level of sleep distortion.

3. If your main complaint is waking too early in the morning, despite no need to be up at that time, (late insomnia) then use the week-long Pre-course Sleep Diary to determine, on average, how long you were awake in the morning before you needed to be up (the difference in minutes, between Question 8 and Question 10). Let's say, on average, you were awake 38 minutes earlier than you needed to be every morning over that week. Also record how many times that week you were above that average. Let's say five times. Now, as with problems getting off to sleep, set an alarm on your phone for 38 minutes earlier than you need to wake up. As before, the alarm should be a single ping and not one that would wake you up should you be asleep at the time. Over the next week, once you have completed your On-course Sleep Diary in the morning, record whether you heard the alarm, or not. At the end of the week determine how far off you were between the number of alarms you heard and the number of times you went over the average from the Pre-course Sleep Diary. That will tell you your level of distortion.

If you have a mixture of sleep complaints, don't try to do all three experiments in one night or indeed one week. Choose one experiment then, once you have determined your level of distortion for that complaint, move on to the next. So, now you have identified how much, on average, you have a sleep distortion. You may now be asking, 'Well that's fine, but how can I sort it out?' What we know is by identifying your level of distortion, yourself, you will automatically start to eliminate it. Additionally, the techniques that you will learn throughout the rest of the course, especially the cognitive distraction techniques (see page 137), will also help by changing your relationship with time when you are in bed.

Day 2 Stimulus Control

Using the On-course Sleep Diary

The On-course Sleep Diary is slightly different to your Pre-course Sleep Diary. The reason for this is that during the course we no longer need the diary to be an assessment of what your sleep pattern looks like; we now need it to tell us how well you are adapting to your personalised sleep plan and where there may be problems or areas for improvement. Even though it is different, it should still be completed every morning between 20 and 40 minutes of waking, just to avoid the influence of sleep inertia.

You will see that most of the first section, 'About Yesterday', is gone, other than the question about unintentional sleep, and the other questions in this section have been replaced by a single question regarding whether a nap was needed or not. The reason for this change is that, and as you will see in the stimulus control section of Day 2, daytime napping is generally discouraged unless absolutely necessary.

The second, third and fourth sections of the diary remain largely the same and we are still recording your main symptoms. You may notice that we are now talking about 'prescribed' time to bed (Question 2) and 'prescribed' time out of bed (Question 7), as opposed to time in and out of bed. Finally, all the sleep variable calculations that you used in the fourth section of the Pre-course Sleep Diary remain the same for the On-course Sleep Diary, although there are now two new additions, Adherence to Prescribed Time to Bed (aPTTB) and Adherence to Prescribed

My Sleep Diary - On-Course

	Day 1	Day 2	Day 3	Day 4	Day 5	Day 6	Day 7	Ave.
About yesterday								
1) Did you unintentionally fall asleep at any point today (yes / no)?								
1a) Did you need to nap today (yes / no)?								
About last night								
2) What time was your prescribed time into bed?								
3) What time did you get into bed?								
4) How long (minutes) did it take you to fall asleep?								
5) If you woke during the night how many times did you wake?								
5a) How long were you awake during the night in total (minutes)?								
About this morning								
6) What time did you wake up (your final awakening)?								
7) How long was this from your prescribed time out of bed (minutes)?								
8) What time did you get out of bed?								
9) How would you rate the quality of your sleep last night (1 = very poor - 5 = excellent)								
10) How refreshed do you feel this morning (1 = not at all - 5 = extremely refreshed)								
Overall								
Prescribed Time In Bed								
Total Duration of Time Awake In Bed								
Total Sleep Time								
Sleep Efficiency %								
Number of Awakenings								
Sleep Latency								
Wake After Sleep Onset								
Adherence to prescribed time in bed								
Adherence to prescribed time out of bed								

Time Out of Bed (aPTOB). The meaning of these two terms will become clearer in a moment.

The next thing to do today is have a look at your first entry on the On-course Sleep Diary (the one you completed this morning). The likelihood is you did not sleep terribly well last night and this is the mild sleep deprivation that I have been talking about. I know it is not nice at all (believe me, I have done this myself and know what it feels like), but please stick with it; it shouldn't last long and it really will pay off in the end.

I like to think of it this way: ask yourself how long you have had insomnia. Let's just say, for argument's sake, two years, as in the case of Lydia (on page 52). That is a maximum of 730 nights of insomnia. Even if Lydia experiences her insomnia at the very minimum (3 nights a week) to qualify as having insomnia, that is still 312 nights of insomnia. Would you be willing to trade a few nights of poor sleep for 312 nights of insomnia? If the answer is yes, great, let's continue. If the answer is no, you may want to reconsider whether the course is right for you, right now or whether having individual face-to-face CBT-I may be more suited to your needs.

The next thing to do with your On-Course Sleep Diary is calculate your Sleep Efficiency (SE), Sleep Latency (SL – the difference, in minutes between Question 6 and Question 8, plus the answer to Question 5a) and Wake After Sleep Onset (WASO the answer to Question 4). Remember your Sleep Efficiency is TST/TIB x 100 (I know I keep repeating this equation, but it really is that essential), although PTIB (Prescribed Time in Bed) replaces the TIB (Time in Bed) in the Pre-course Diary.

Your SE should have increased quite a bit. If it has not, there are two possible explanations: your calculations may be a bit off and I would go back and re-run your numbers just to make sure, or you may be having a bit of trouble following your personal sleep plan.

Adherence

Now let's calculate and examine the last two items of the On-course Sleep Diary which are Adherence to Prescribed Time To Bed (aPTTB) and Adherence to Prescribed Time Out of Bed (aPTOB). For the first item you need to record, in minutes, the difference plus or minus between your Prescribed Time to Bed (Question 2) and your answer to Question 3 – what time you actually went to bed. For example, if my PTTB is 1.30am and I went to bed at 1.15am my aPTTB would be – 15 (minutes).

If everything is working to schedule, this number should be 0. The higher the number, whether it be a plus or a minus, the more we need to address adherence. If there is a plus number you need to ask yourself what is preventing you from going to bed at your prescribed bedtime. If it is a case of losing track of time, that is okay, but you might want to think of ways to reduce that number tonight so you get the full amount of time in bed that you have been prescribed. Otherwise you are depriving yourself of sleep unnecessarily.

What if the number is a minus? Well, that indicates that you went to bed earlier than you were prescribed to do, as in our example, and we need to determine, and address, the reasons for this. Was it that you were tired and felt that you needed to go to bed? Was it just habit? Either way, going to bed earlier than your PTTB is going to result in a watered-down version of sleep rescheduling, which is not good and you are not likely to improve your sleep that much.

The same is true if your adherence to the Prescribed Time Out of Bed – which is the difference, in minutes, between Question 8 and your PTOB (Question 7) – is a positive number. Again, you should be aiming for 0. If it is a minus number, you are not using all the allotted time in bed (again, increasing your levels of sleep deprivation unnecessarily) but if it is a plus number, you are staying in bed when you should have been out of the bed (again, a watered-down version of sleep rescheduling). I would love to say it does not matter that much, but I am afraid it really does matter. You are not going to see the full benefits of the course if you don't stick to both your Prescribed Time to Bed and Prescribed Time Out of Bed.

Stimulus Control

This aspect of the course was created by Professor Richard (Dick) Bootzin and here we are going to be dealing with any conditioned arousal that may have developed. As we saw on page 57, the constant pairing of the bedroom and/or pre-sleep routine with not being able to sleep can result in waking you up and making you feel more alert at bedtime. Even thinking about the bedroom can now elicit negative thoughts, feelings and emotions. Interestingly, it does not end there. The more 'activities' (reading, watching television, listening to the radio) we do in the bedroom, in order to 'help' us sleep or to compensate for the time being awake in the night, the more likely those activities will also become conditioned stimuli to being awake at night, given enough pairings. When you were a normal sleeper those activities were not likely to be associated with being awake, as sleep came whether you did the activity or not. Now, the situation is different and so we need to take a different approach.

On page 56 I talked about my own conditioned response to snacking in my office. In order to break that associa-tion (and save myself from putting on even more weight), I stopped snacking in my office and forced myself to go to the dining room to eat whenever I was hungry. That was my form of stimulus control. In terms of sleep, stimulus control has two main parts; the first is about eliminating all the negative conditioned stimuli that exist between your bed and being awake and the second is about reconditioning a positive association between bedroom/bed and sleep. Here are the rules:

1. Only use the bedroom for sleep or sex, and no sleeping elsewhere (including napping)
2. If you are in bed and not asleep and you get to the point that you know that sleep is not going to happen (at any point during the night), get out of the bed and leave the bedroom (if possible and practical).

In terms of the first rule, we are eliminating every other possible conditioned stimulus from the bedroom environment, except sex, which is good for sleep anyway. Additionally, by doing this, coupled with the sleep rescheduling, we are increasing the chances of the pairing of bed and sleep as opposed to bed and wake activities (reading, watching TV, listening to music). The reason for not sleeping anywhere else is about sending ourselves mixed messages about where you can sleep and thus reducing the strength of the conditioned response we are aiming for (bed = sleep). Additionally, as I have said before, napping (unless absolutely necessary) disrupts the sleep homeostat.

You may have heard a version of the second rule called 'the 15-minute rule'. According to this version, if you are not asleep within 15 minutes of getting into bed or if you are awake for more than 15 minutes in the night you should get up and leave the bedroom. The reason I have modified this slightly is the issue of how do you know when 15 minutes is up and you have to leave the bedroom? I have already asked you to remove visible clocks from the bedroom, as part of your sleep hygiene, so the '15-minute rule' sounds a little contradictory. Besides, who says it has to be 15 minutes exactly? In essence, what I am trying to do here is avoid you getting angry, frustrated or miserable in bed; in other words, reinforcing any conditioned arousal to the bed and bedroom. In my experience, there is a point at which, just before we get angry, frustrated or miserable, that we know that sleep is not coming and that for me is the time for action.

The first question I usually get is, 'What am I going to do when I get out of bed and leave the bedroom?' Here it is all about planning. In terms of the activities you can do, the exact same rules apply as for the period of time before your Prescribed Time to Bed (PTTB) on page 116. Anything you like except napping, pornography, work, a meal, exercise, blue light, and as long as it is safe and not going to cause harm to you or disruption to others.

What I would say here is that it can be quite a challenge to get out of a nice, warm, cosy bed. One way to manage this is to identify and set up a space where you plan to go, before you go to bed. Make sure the space is warm (not hot), has enough light for you to do whatever activity you choose to do and that you have everything ready to do the chosen activity. The one thing I do usually suggest is to avoid reclining on the sofa or on a comfy chair as you are likely to fall asleep there and that is not what we want, as I mentioned in Day 1 when we talked about sleep rescheduling. Additionally, remember the first rule, no sleeping elsewhere, as we want the pairing of bed = sleep not sofa = sleep.

The other question I get a lot at this point is, 'Is it not better for me to stay in bed as at least I will be resting?' The answer to this is no. On page 14 we talked about the sleep homeostat and the impact even small naps can have. The same thing applies here. Even a small amount of waxing and waning in and out of sleep (Dr Michael Perlis calls this 'sleep surfing') is going to reduce your overall drive to sleep and if this waxing and waning pattern happens during bedtime, that is going to keep you awake a great deal longer.

The final thing to consider is when do you go back to the bedroom? Again, there are two schools of thought: go back to bed only when you are sleepy or determine an amount of time to be out of bed beforehand and only go back to bed when your time is up.

Previously I was an advocate of the former strategy as I felt that would be less disruptive than setting a specific period of time before you went back to bed. Recently, however, I have come to change my mind about this and now suggest that you set yourself an amount of time to be awake before going back to bed, either 30 minutes or 45 minutes. In my recent experience, believe it or not, this latter strategy is the less disruptive of the two. So, why 30 or 45 minutes? They are the average lengths of a sit-com episode or episode of a television series without adverts. This makes it very easy to manage knowing when it is time to go back to bed.

The final part of this aspect of stimulus control is to repeat this process as many times as necessary. In other words, if you go back to bed after being out for 30 or 45 minutes and, again, you get to that point of knowing that sleep is not going to happen, get out of bed again for another 30 or 45 minutes. Repeat this as many times as is necessary throughout the whole period between PTTB and PTOB.

Along those lines, the other thing I get asked about at this point is whether you should just give up going back to bed in the later hours of the morning. If, for example, your PTOB is 7am, should you go back to bed for 15 minutes if your last period of being out of bed (i.e. when your programme finishes) is at 6.45am. My answer is yes, go back to bed but don't stay in bed beyond your PTOB (in this case 7am).

Finally, you may be wondering how we are going to address the conditioned arousal to the pre-sleep routine, as in Lydia's case (see page 55). To be perfectly honest, the sleep rescheduling and stimulus control techniques combined should take care of that as you should be really tired by the time you go to bed under your personalised sleep plan. That said, it couldn't hurt to switch your pre-sleep routine around a little bit if you feel it would add anything. Lydia did; she started brushing her teeth after dinner as opposed to right before she was going to bed. Whether that change added anything to her treatment or whether it was the combination of that, the sleep rescheduling and the stimulus control I could not tell you, but it worked overall and she no longer gets those feelings of stress, anxiety and wakefulness when she goes to bed.

Alternatives to Leaving the Bedroom at Night

It may be impractical or impossible for you to leave the bedroom while doing stimulus control. You may live in a studio apartment, for example, or in an environment where leaving the bedroom is likely to disrupt other people (caregiving is a good example here). What can we do in these circumstances?

I would still prefer you to get out of the bed, so for now that is a given. Instead, set aside a specific space in the bedroom for you to go to during those times out of bed. Call it your 'wake zone' as opposed to your 'sleep zone' (the bed). If you have to get out of the bed as you have got to the point that you know that sleep is not happening, get out and go to the 'wake zone'. The same rules as above will apply in terms of activities you can do in the wake zone, when it is time to go back to bed (after 30 or 45 minutes) and repeating the process as necessary.

I also remember a case where an individual had to travel for work while she was going to be introducing stimulus control into her personalised sleep plan and during this time she would be staying in a hotel. She asked me whether she should post-pone doing this part of the course until she was back home. My response was no. Hotels tend to have a lobby. Either that, or if you feel slightly uncomfortable about being in the lobby of a hotel during the night (which I actually find is a fascinat-ing thing to do if I am practising stimulus control when I am away ... yes, I still do stimulus control when necessary), then set up a 'wake zone' in your hotel room.

Alternatives to Leaving the Bed at Night

While none of the other activities that we have suggested in this section should change, I do appreciate that for some people there may be an issue with getting out of the bed during the night. This is not to be taken as an excuse not to get out of bed because you did not want to but, rather, where circumstances suggest it is impractical or impossible to get out of the bed.

These circumstances mainly include those individuals who may have mobility issues, sight issues (considering the requisite for darkness in the bedroom) or those who are vulnerable to falls.

I have come across three rather different scenarios where getting out of the bed at night was not an option – a patient who was paralysed, a CBT-I study Dr Zoe Gotts, Professor Julia Newton, Dr Vincent Deary and I conducted on patients with severe Chronic Fatigue Syndrome/ME, and, most recently, a colleague, Charlotte Randall, and I conducted a study using a brief form of CBT-I, shorter than this one, believe it or not, in a group of male prisoners. In each case, getting out of bed was not really an option, let alone leaving the room altogether. In these instances, I created a modified approach to stimulus control, which has worked pretty well in each case. Everything remains the same. In other words, instigate the stimulus control at the point you realise that you are not likely to sleep and just before you start getting frustrated, angry or miserable but, instead of getting out of the bed, you move to the other side of the bed or, if appropriate, get your carers to move you to the other side of the bed. In this case, you have designated one side of the bed for sleeping and one side of the bed for being awake. You can do any of the activities listed earlier (if able) on the 'wake' side of the bed, for the predetermined time (30 or 45 minutes), and then back over to the 'sleep' side of the bed. Finally, as before, repeat if necessary.

Day 3 Cognitive Control

So, first things first: let's examine your On-course Sleep Diary from this morning. After two nights on your new sleep routine you are still likely to feel tired and maybe a little more irritable than usual. The first thing to say is that this is perfectly normal. It is not that the sleep rescheduling is not working; in fact, quite the opposite – it is a sign that it is working. Again, please stick with it, it will get better and you will feel less sleepy and irritable in a day or so. It is just taking a little time for your body to readjust to your personalised sleep plan.

One of the things I do here, at least when I am seeing someone face-to-face, is tell him or her to call my office answerphone (naturally, I am not going to give out my home phone number or mobile) if they like and leave a message telling me exactly what they think about me and their treatment. People have said it helps. What you may want to do, as I am not giving everyone reading this my office number, is use your time out of bed to write me a long letter telling me what you think about the course so far. You don't have to post it, and I am not promising to write back, but it may indeed help.

Now, what you may well notice from your On-course Sleep Diary is that the time it takes you to fall asleep (Sleep Latency) and the amount of time you are awake at night (Wake After Sleep Onset) have already started to reduce a little over the last two days, but we will look more carefully at those tomorrow when we have a clearer picture. More importantly, what we do know is that the sleep that you are getting now, even after just two days, is going to be deeper and more consolidated. Remember to calculate your adherence numbers (aPTTB and aPTOB) again and, if there is a disparity still, in either direction, plus or minus, start to think about ways you can manage what is preventing you from sticking to your PTTB and PTOB. Please don't change your PTIB or indeed your PTTB or PTOB, however tempting that may be, as any benefits you have already gained, including this adaptation time, will be lost if you do.

Before we leave the On-course Sleep Diary for today, I want to discuss the answer to Questions 1 and 1a. Remember, this is about NEEDING a nap, not wanting a nap, which you may want to do. If you answered yes to either question, that is a red flag and we need to re-evaluate our position. It is not normal for someone with insomnia, even while doing sleep rescheduling and stimulus control, to need a nap or unintentionally fall asleep two days into the treatment. If this is the case, DO NOT continue with sleep rescheduling or stimulus control. Make an appointment to see a Behavioural Sleep Medicine specialist. Explain to them what you have been doing and specifically that there has been a significant increase in your daytime sleepiness to the point of needing to nap or falling asleep unintentionally. If they are BSMs worth their salt, they will understand that this is not usual and will arrange a series of tests to see whether there is an underlying issue or other illness or condition that you may be unaware of that needs some attention before you can continue. In these cases remember to go back to the algorithm and complete the Pre-course Sleep Diary before re-starting the course when, and if, you come back to the course.

Putting the Day to Bed Before You Go to Bed

Right, let's start cognitive control. This is the first cognitive element of the course and it is designed both to reduce your racing mind and help you manage worry so they don't impact on your sleep at night. I like to refer to this part of the course as putting the day to bed before you go to bed. It certainly is not as arduous as sleep rescheduling and stimulus control and people tend to like doing this technique.

The first part of this technique is determining a cut-off time. This is the point at which you need to stop all your daytime activities, such as work. After dinner, or supper, tends to be a natural break in the evening, which, if you are making sure you are not eating within 2 hours of bedtime, leaves you plenty of separation between the day and the night. A lot of people do this naturally, but try to stick to this time, however tempting it is to do a little more paperwork or email after your meal.

Your Cognitive Control Diary

What we will need for the second part of cognitive control is a notebook and a pen. This may sound odd, but if you can get a notebook with a cover that would be great. The reason for this will become apparent in a moment. The main reason for doing cognitive control is because, when we are awake at night, we tend to use this time to think and those thoughts usually start out with a review of the day's events, then progress on to things we have to do tomorrow and then on to thinking, and worrying, about bigger, broader issues. Remember Lydia? She would do exactly that, in that same order, when she got into bed and could not sleep. This technique is intended to combat that and leave you feeling as if you are more in control of your day, which will translate into less worry and less to think about at night.

This activity should be completed at least 2 hours before your prescribed bedtime. Set yourself about 45 minutes to an hour to do this. There are two parts to this technique. The first part deals with your short-term thoughts (today and tomorrow). So you need to create a series of four lists in your notebook. The headings for the four lists should be as follows:

1. Everything that I have accomplished today
2. Everything that I have to achieve tomorrow
3. Everything that I have put into place to deal with tomorrow
4. A few lines on how I feel about how my day went (your emotional state).

Everything that I have accomplished today	How I feel about how my day went
Completed this template	Actually the day did not go too badly. I feel more in control and I know that things will work out tomorrow at the meeting, although I am a bit nervous, as I have sorted everything that I can think of. I was a bit upset that I did not find time to do the letter for Celyne straightaway but, if I use the template from the last letter I wrote, that should be fine.
Finished writing book chapter	
Completed paperwork for NHS	
Ordered Harry's medication	
Organised train to London for next week	
Created teaching materials for start of semester	

	Everything that I have to do/achieve tomorrow	Everything that I have put into place to deal with tomorrow
1	Meeting with Dean of Faculty	Got paperwork ready to sign, on desk
2	Coffee with Martin at the University	Set alarm clock
3	Review grant proposal	Printed off, ready to read
4	Call my brother	
5	Food shopping	List is on the fridge
6	Sort out dinner with Zoe for next week	
7	Send book chapter to Susan	All ready, in the book file on my laptop
8	Write letter for Celyne	I have a template to use in my office
9	Arrange Skype with Michael (email)	
10	Go to bank	
11	Organise meeting with Pam	
12	Organise online reading lists for students	List is on my desk
13	Co-ordinate dates to see Annette	
14	Finish writing for Pain Conference in Holland	Printed out Carla's comments on my draft
15	Call mother	Bite the bullet on that one

On page 132, I have provided an example of a Cognitive Control Diary to show you how I do it. Although the choice of format is entirely up to you, as you may have your own preference for the order or style in which you write them down, it is important that you cover all four elements. Additionally, this should not be just one quick pass-over. Think about it, come back to a heading and keep adding to it. Hence why you have about 20–30 minutes to do this part. I am not suggesting that you should be racking your brain to remember whether you had a biscuit at 11am, or not, but it should be a comprehensive overview of your main activities.

The second part of this strategy is constructive worry time and you should devote about 20 minutes to this part. I want you to create a table with three columns. Again, I have provided an example below.

In the first column (labelled 'Worry or concern') I want you to write down your biggest worries and concerns that are NOT related to your sleep or insomnia (we will deal with sleep- and insomnia-related worries and concerns later on page 143). In the second column (labelled 'What can I do about that situation right now?') you can put one of three options here: nothing at all/nothing comes to mind (red), nothing right now but later (yellow) or something immediate (green). In the third column (labelled 'Actions') write down as many possible solutions or ways forward as you can think of alongside all of the yellow and green responses. If you have a red response, where there is no action that you can think of right now, leave that part of the action column blank. Finally, review your solutions, and transfer any that you feel you could implement tomorrow to part 2 ('Everything I have to do/achieve tomorrow') of your Cognitive Control Diary. I have provided an example below.

	Worry or concern	What can I do about that situation right now?		Action(s)
1	I am not going to finish reviewing the grant by the deadline	GREEN	1	Cancel my trip now so I can work on the review
			2	
2	Janet says she hates Susan because Susan said some unkind things about her	YELLOW	1	Talk to Janet tomorrow
			2	Talk to Susan tomorrow
3	Bobby at work has accepted a new job and will be leaving	RED	1	
			2	
4	I forgot to leave a note for Jackie	GREEN	1	Text her now instead
			2	
5	Sam did not get his promotion	YELLOW	1	Meet with him next week to talk about his next application
			2	Read the reviews as to why he did not get promoted
6			1	
			2	
7			1	
			2	
8			1	
			2	

RED = Nothing at all/nothing comes to mind
YELLOW = Nothing right now, but later
GREEN = Something immediate

Once you have completed all the sections in your notebook, I want you to close the cover and place it by the bed, with the pen. Closing the cover is a symbolic gesture that tells us that the day has been put to bed and, believe it or not, it is actually beneficial. If, during the night, you do start to think about something that needs to be done tomorrow, you now know, and can remind yourself, that you already have it covered in the notebook. If, on the other hand, you think of something that you had previously forgotten, then you have the notebook and pen by the bed and so you can jot it down, close the notebook again, and tell yourself it is done with for tonight. The great thing about this technique is it is cumulative and you can transfer things from the lists from one day to the next if you don't get them done in time.

Day 4 Cognitive Distraction Techniques

As always, we start with your On-course Sleep Diary. You should have now completed three nights of sleep rescheduling, two nights of stimulus control and one night of cognitive control. At this point your body should be starting to adjust to your personalised sleep plan and the morning sleepiness that you have been experiencing should be starting to go away. In most cases it will not have gone away completely but should have reduced somewhat. Remember what I said yesterday about the answers to Questions 1 and 1a? If you answer yes, this indicates (even more so than yesterday) that something needs attention and you should STOP sleep rescheduling and stimulus control and arrange to see a Behavioural Sleep Medicine specialist.

Now, let's look at your symptoms. Compare your average Sleep Latency (SL) and Wake After Sleep Onset (WASO), from your Pre-course Sleep Diary with your SL and WASO from this morning's On-course Sleep Diary. Also compare your average Sleep Efficiency (SE) from the Pre-course Sleep Diary with this morning's Sleep Efficiency. All things considered, you should be seeing some improvements. Specifically, your SE should have increased and your SL and WASO decreased.

If your problem was predominantly one of getting off to sleep, you will probably see a bigger improvement than if your problem was predominantly one of waking up during the night or in the early morning. Why sleep rescheduling and stimulus control have a bigger impact on SL before WASO at this point, we are not entirely sure, but this is generally how it works. If you are not seeing a significant drop in your WASO, please don't worry – it will continue to drop as you progress. The other thing to remember is that this is just the beginning; both SL and WASO should continue to drop as we go forward. In terms of your SE, this should have increased significantly. If it has not, the first thing to do is check your calculations to make sure they are accurate. The reason I am saying that is, by the very nature of sleep rescheduling, which eliminates any time in bed that you are awake, your SE should increase significantly as SE assesses the difference between Time Awake in Bed and Total Sleep Time. Finally, calculate your adherence measures and hopefully we should be at, or at least very close to, 0. If it is not, you may have to really consider if the course is right for you, right now, as without adherence to the sleep rescheduling and stimulus control you are not going to see the full benefits of this course. If this is the case it may be worth seeking out a BSM for individual face-to-face CBT-I.

Cognitive Distraction

At this point we are going to add another technique, which fits perfectly on top of cognitive control. Here we are going to deal with the racing mind while you are in bed. This will account for not only the racing mind while getting off to sleep, but also the racing mind if we wake up in the night or early morning. In essence, with cognitive control we have given you more control over your day and reduced the capacity for a racing mind at night because of short-term and longer-term worries and concerns. The difficulty with cognitive control, as a stand-alone technique, is that if we have an empty mind at night and we are awake, we are likely to fill it with something else and it is likely to be negative and related to our sleep. The thing that we need to do here is fill the mind so that those negative, sleep-related, or indeed, other-related, thoughts cannot occur. We do this by giving you something else to concentrate on. This, as a by-product, also helps with reducing sleep effort, as you will have enough to think about. So, we need to find something that is all consuming to the mind but contains no emotion whatsoever.

Here I am going to introduce you to three strategies that we can use to achieve that goal. Why three? Well, we are all different and, in my experience, people tend to have a preference for one of three types of cognitive distraction strategy – numeric, alphabetical or visual – over the other two. I am going to give you all three strategies and then you can decide based upon your preferences, or through a process of trial and error, which is the most beneficial for you.

The one thing I would say here is to be mindful about any crossover between whichever strategy you choose and elements from your day-to-day life. For example, if you work with numbers all day (if you are an accountant, say) you should probably NOT choose to do the number technique as you may find yourself inadvertently thinking about work. Similarly, if you are a travel agent, pilot or member of aircrew you probably would NOT choose cities of the world if you were looking to do an alphabet-based distraction technique, for the same reason. This will become clearer as we go through each strategy.

Numeric

I am sure you have heard about counting sheep to help you sleep and some of you may have already tried it, with, I am guessing, very limited success. The thing to think about here is that counting is the right thing to do in principle (it is distracting) but the problem is that counting sheep is just too simple a task. I can be watching Flossy the sheep jumping over a fence, in my mind's eye, while thinking about how I am going to pay the mortgage this month at the same time. What we need here is something a little more taxing or consuming. So, instead of counting sheep (one sheep, two sheep, three sheep, etc.), I am going to ask you to count backwards, from one thousand in sevens (so, one thousand, nine hundred and ninety-three, nine hundred and eighty-six, nine hundred and seventy-nine, etc.). Sounds tough, right? It is meant to be.

The beauty of this technique is that I am not bothered whether you get the numbers right or whether you lose your place; it is all about being mentally consumed by it. So, what happens if you get a number wrong or lose your place? Just start again. The question I get here is, 'For how long should I do this, or any of these cognitive distraction strategies for that matter?' Here, I go back to the stimulus control rule (see page 124). As soon as you get to the point that you know that sleep is not going to happen, stop doing the strategy and get out of the bed. In my experience, however, people don't tend to get that far. It is almost as if, and this is a study yet to be done, the brain has reached either a point of overload or an extreme level of boredom, and sleep is the desired alternative.

Alphabetical

The same principle applies to the alphabetical strategy; we are just changing the focus from numbers to words. A patient gave the following example to me a few years ago and I absolutely love it and always use it now. He suggested that you play a game, one that I think most of us have played or at least know of.

Firstly, choose a category; let's say cities of the world. Start with a city, say, Amsterdam. Amsterdam ends with the letter M, so now I need to think of a city that starts with M, say, Madrid. Madrid ends in D, so Düsseldorf and on we go. Over the years people have chosen alternative categories (animals, foods, colours, clothing); just make sure there are lots of choice options as it is not going to help if you choose a very narrow category, such as airlines, for example. Others have changed the rules of the game slightly; such as naming all foods you can think of that begin with A, then B, then C, etc. Either way is fine, as long as it is mentally consuming and not emotionally provocative.

This is one of the main areas where your day-to-day life may influence how well this strategy works for you. For the alphabetical technique I said that people who work in the travel industry should avoid cities of the world; here, greengrocers should probably avoid fruit and vegetable categories, and so forth.

Visual

I will be honest, this is my least favourite distraction technique, but I have included it because some people really like it and say that it works for them.

As with the alphabetical strategy start with a category. Let's say fruit. What is your favourite fruit? I love mango (I am not allowed to use rhubarb, which would have been my first choice, as it is a vegetable, apparently). I want you to imagine the most perfect mango, one where the skin starts out at the bottom end a shiny green, then blends into a pale yellow which then fades into a shiny red. The stalk is small and brown peeking out from the top and there is one shiny green leaf attached to the mango. Once you have the mango absolutely picture perfect in your mind, including shade, colour and dimensions, then you need to mentally turn the mango blue. Now that your mango is predominantly blue, you have to determine, in your head, what colours, shades and dimension the rest of the mango is going to be. What colour is the stalk now, what about the leaf? I hope you can see where this is going. Once your blue mango is complete, turn it orange and so forth.

Day 5 Decatastrophising Sleep

Let's start with your Sleep Diary calculations, as always. We need to look specifically at Questions 1 and 1a, as we do every day, and, if you answer yes to either, then we need to stop everything and see a Behavioural Sleep Medicine specialist. Now, I am not going to go on and on about your adherence figures; that is for you to determine whether there is an issue here, and address, or not.

On to decatastrophising sleep. This is my favourite technique and I apply it to many different areas in my life, not just in relation to sleep. The reason I talk about decatastrophising is simple: we all tend to catastrophise to some degree or another but this can become quite problematic for someone with insomnia.

So, what do we mean by catastrophising? In the context of sleep and insomnia, it is a tendency to become overly preoccupied with our sleep with a negative interpretation. Lydia talked about dwelling on the topic of sleep 'almost all the time' (see page 54). That is definitely evidence of sleep preoccupation, which is not great on its own, but the catastrophising part is when we assign overly negative interpretations alongside this preoccupation. Think of it this way, Lydia clearly has quite high levels of sleep preoccupation but also feels that her insomnia is likely to make her very, very ill in the long term. That last part is a sign of sleep catastrophising.

Where I have done quite a bit of research myself in the area of sleep preoccupation, which I have incorporated into my version of CBT-I, I have to say that Professor Allison Harvey has done much of the work in terms of sleep catastrophising.

Where sleep catastrophising becomes, in my view, even more of an interesting and important issue is that it appears that catastrophising during the night is not quite the same thing as catastrophising during the day for most of us, with catastrophising at night being much more likely to occur, unrealistic in content and more negatively focused. This actually makes some sense. Think about the beginning of the book when I talked about normal sleep and the different stages of sleep (page 20). I mentioned that different parts of the brain are down-regulated over the whole process of sleep whereas different parts of the brain are more or less affected by down-regulation during the different stages of sleep. The thing to note here is, even though an individual may be awake at night, some of those parts of the brain that would be down-regulating if we were asleep are still down-regulating at that time even though we are awake.

One of those areas of the brain that is down-regulated during the night, irrespective of whether we are asleep or awake, is the part of the brain that covers rationality, reasoning and logic. As such, we may be awake but our ability to think logically and rationally is, for want of a better term, asleep. This can make even the simplest issue or event appear even more catastrophic at night.

A good example of this difference between daytime catastrophising and night-time catastrophising came from Mary, a really nice woman whom I was seeing for her insomnia quite a while back. I asked Mary what she thought about at night when she was awake and she had a wonderful response, 'Last night it was the dishwasher ... believe me ... the bloody dishwasher ... I was there at two o'clock in the morning worrying about whether the leak I had cleared up earlier in the day was a sign that the dishwasher was on its last legs. Then I started to worry about how I was going to arrange getting it fixed ... then how I would manage without it ... then the cost of a new one.' She went on to say, 'The next morning the first thing I remembered was the dishwasher ... so I got it looked at ... there was no problem ... end of.' You can see that Mary recognised, during the day, that she was thinking catastrophically at night but was unable to stop herself from doing it.

The thing here is that you are probably not going to be able to stop yourself from catastrophising at night. If I wanted to stop doing it altogether, I would either not leave an opportunity for it to happen; in other words sleep through the night (this is another reason why sleep rescheduling and stimulus control have been introduced first this week), or I would have to wake up fully at that time and that is not what we really want to do. So, here I am going to teach you how to manage this, if it happens, instead. What I would stress is that this technique is NOT there to minimise the consequences of your insomnia but rather highlight disproportionate catastrophic thinking at night.

Managing Catastrophising

This is a technique that should be done in the daytime. You will need a pen and pad and definitely a calculator (unless you are really good at maths) for this one. I want you to think about those times in the night that you are awake and specifically thinking about the consequences of your insomnia (both short term and long term). Here I want your worst-case scenario. How do we get to that? I will show you with some dialogue between a patient, Val, and myself:

Me – Okay, so you are up in the night, what goes through your mind?

Val – Well, my immediate thought is I am not going to get any sleep tonight.

Me – Right, and what does that mean to you in terms of consequences the next day?

Val – I am not going to have a good day at work.

Me – And? If you don't have a good day at work, what does that ultimately mean? Worst-case scenario.

Val – I am going to get a warning for not reaching my targets.

Me – And then?

Val – Well, ultimately they will get rid of me.

Me – You mean fired, right? Not killed.

Val – Yes, fired ... not that sort of organisation [laugh].

Me – Okay, so you lose your job, then what?

Val – Well, I'm 56 ... you know ... so I don't think I'll get another job ... at least not at that level ... and not that pay.

Me – And what are the consequences of not having another job at that level?

Val – I won't be able to afford my house.

Me – And? If you can't afford your house?

Val – I don't know ... I will be evicted ... there you go ... worst-case scenario. I will end up on the streets [laugh].

Now, I know what I have done here with Val seems a little bit contrived but let's think about it this way: during the daytime, yes, it is contrived, but we are trying to get to those illogical, irrational catastrophic thoughts that tend to happen at night when that part of our brain is asleep. I want you to now imagine that you and I are having that same dialogue – what would be your three worst-case scenarios? List them on a piece of paper (use my template below, if that helps).

People usually get to events such as crashing their car, a serious illness, losing a job or divorce. Then I ask, 'With what percentage of certainty, at night, do you think that event (for example, losing a job) is going to happen?' Remember, this is your estimate during the night, not during the day when you are thinking more realistically. Let's carry on with Val. She reported a 70% feeling of certainty that she would lose her job, because of her insomnia, when she was awake in the middle of the night. So, in a column next to each of the three worst-case scenarios work out what percentage, at night, you believe that each event is going to happen.

Catastrophic event	% I believe, at night, this will happen	Length of insomnia in nights*	How many times should this have happened**	How many times this has actually happened	% of times this has happened***	Comparison to remember at night	
						Night	Day
Going to crash my car as I am so tired	90%	2.5 years for 3 nights a week = 391 nights	90/100 x 391 = 352 times	0	0%	90%	0%
Going to get diabetes	40%	2.5 years for 3 nights a week = 391 nights	40/100 x 391 = 156 times	0	0%	40%	0%
Going to ruin my relationship	70%	2.5 years for 3 nights a week = 391 nights	70/100 x 391 = 273 times	2 (possibly)	0.26%	70%	0.26%

* Number of nights with insomnia divided by 7, multiplied by the number of nights a week, on average, affected
** % I believe will happen divided by 100, multiplied by length of insomnia in nights
*** Number of times happened divided by number of nights of insomnia, multiplied by 100

The next thing I usually do is work out how long you have had insomnia. In Val's case it had been around 11 years (maximum 4,015 nights). As we know, insomnia tends not to happen every night so on average how many nights of insomnia do you experience in a typical week? For Val, her best guess was about 4 nights a week, on average. So that would be (4,015 / 7) x 4 = 2,294 nights of insomnia. So, if Val is 70% (70/100) sure of losing her job on 2,294 nights of insomnia (0.7 x 2,294), and if this were a rational and logical thought, she should have lost her job on 1,606 occasions (I have rounded up the .8 at the end in case you were wondering).

Now you need to do the same calculations and work out how many times each of the worst-case scenarios that you have identified should have happened to you over the time that you have had your insomnia if these were rational daytime thoughts.

Next we need to find out what is happening in reality. So how many times has Val actually lost her job because of her 11 years of insomnia? The answer was none, or perhaps once, although she could not be certain that it was because of her insomnia that she lost that particular job as a lot of other things were going on at the time.

For argument's sake, let's take this as one time, even though there is some doubt there about the cause, so in the 11 years or 2,294 nights of insomnia that Val has had, the actual number of times this worst-case scenario has happened was once or, turning that to a percentage, the actual chances of this occurring were (1/2,294) or 0.0004%. So, we have an actual daytime occurrence of 0.0004% versus a belief, during the night, that it will occur of 70% of the time. The difference between these numbers is good evidence of some sleep-related catastrophic thinking going on.

Now you need to do the same. Work out how many times the actual worst-case scenario has actually occurred; remember it only counts if you believe the event was a direct result of your insomnia. Divide that number by the number of nights of insomnia you have had and write that in the next column. The difference between those two percentages is your level of nocturnal catastrophic thinking.

The last thing we need to do is translate that back into your night. If you are awake at night and you start thinking about the awful consequences of insomnia (for example, losing your job) go back to your calculations (in Val's case, 0.0004%) and keep telling yourself something like 'my reason sleeps elsewhere'.

Day 6 Sleep Titration and Progressive Muscle Relaxation

By now you should know the drill. Sleep Diary first. However, all I really want to concentrate on today is your Sleep Efficiency. That is not to say that all the other variables that you have been dealing with (SL, WASO, Adherence numbers) are irrelevant, as these should be calculated also, but we are going to use your average Sleep Efficiency, since starting the course, to start titrating you. Remember, we will NOT be doing this if you have Paradoxical Insomnia.

What Do We Mean By Titration?

In essence, we are going to check whether your original Prescribed Time in Bed (PTIB) from the Pre-course Sleep Diary needs increasing or reducing or, indeed, whether it needs to stay the same.

One of the difficulties with CBT-I, and this course included, is that I did not know what your actual sleep need was when we first started and we now need to start adjusting your personal sleep plan to what your sleep need is. So, at the beginning, when we calculated your Prescribed Time in Bed we used the average amount of time you slept during the pre-course period (i.e. your Total Sleep Time) as a gross indicator. We are going to determine how far off you are from your sleep need and start moving in that direction. How do we do this? Well, we will increase, decrease or keep your PTIB the same, based upon a set of titration rules.

The Rules of Titration

The way I like to describe the rules of titration is through the analogy of a card game, something like blackjack or pontoon. When you are playing these types of games you tend to have three options depending upon the cards you are holding (Twist, Stick or Bust). Twist is when you do not have enough points in your hand so you need an additional card. Stick is when you have enough points in your hand so you stay where you are and Bust is when you already have too many points and are over the limit (and if you could, although it may be cheating in the context of a card game, you would give a card, or two, away).

The hand you hold represents your Sleep Efficiency from the On-course Sleep Diary that you have been completing every morning and here a rule of plus or minus 15 minutes relates to what you need to do next.

For younger adults (18 to 65 years old) without any illness or medication complications, if you are, from the average over the last 5 days, under 85% Sleep Efficiency then you Twist and take 15 minutes away from your PTIB. If you are 85–90% Sleep Efficiency then you Stick and don't do anything with your PTIB. If you are above 90% Sleep Efficiency, then you have Bust and add 15 minutes to your existing PTIB.

For older adults (65 years or older) or those who have illness or medication complications we have slightly different rules to account for age-related changes in your sleep need (see page 28) and illness- or medication-related factors. In these instances if you have an average, over the last 5 days, Sleep Efficiency below 80% you Twist, 80–85% you Stick and above 85% you Bust. In the case of Twist and Bust you will still be working with 15 minutes.

The 5-hour minimum rule (discussed on page 110) is also still in effect, and should always be, so, if your Sleep Efficiency suggests that you should take 15 minutes away from your PTIB (i.e. Twist), but you are already at 5 hours' PTIB you should stay at 5 hours and NOT go to 4¾ hours.

Why 15 minutes? The reason for this is that it appears to be just the right balance between giving someone too much time back and possibly worsening their Sleep Efficiency, and taking too much time away, which may cause a big jump in terms of sleep deprivation. Some people have suggested bigger levels of titration, such as 30 or even 45 minutes, but I completely disagree with doing that as I feel that 15 minutes is a safe titration limit. The other thing to remember here is the anchor time (your Prescribed Time Out of Bed) stays the same, so you only add or subtract 15 minutes from your Prescribed Time to Bed.

The next question people ask is how often should they titrate. Under a full six–eight-week programme of CBT-I I would say at the end of each week and, for the purposes of this course, I would say exactly the same from here on in. So, at this point you may be saying, 'Hang on, is the course not nearly finished?' The answer, in the main, is yes. You still have managing success and relapse prevention to do but everything else is now in your hands and you have all the necessary tools to get to your ideal Sleep Efficiency. In my experience, people do not have to titrate every week for the full six–eight weeks to reach a good sleep efficiency goal as they will have reached it (ideally, for younger adults without illness or medication use between 85–90% Sleep Efficiency and for older adults or those with an illness or medication use between 80–85% Sleep Efficiency) well before then.

A final thing I get asked at this point is, 'Why I am not aiming for a Sleep Efficiency goal of 100%?' It's a good question and the reason for this is that even good sleepers, let alone 'normal' sleepers, still take a little time to fall asleep and may, on occasion, spend a small amount of time awake during the night. A perfect, or near perfect, Sleep Efficiency, is to me an indicator that you are a little sleep deprived and that is why we set the limits as they are. The key point here is getting to your Sleep Efficiency optimum limit while asking yourself how you feel in the morning (at least 20 minutes after you have awoken, see page 97). You will know when you have reached your optimum, and this is generally when you have high Sleep Efficiency levels and also wake up in the morning feeling alert and refreshed. That is why I have included measures of sleep quality and feelings of being refreshed in the morning on the Pre-Course and On-Course Sleep Diaries. That, in my view; should be your Sleep Efficiency goal.

Progressive Muscle Relaxation

Progressive Muscle Relaxation, which has been around for over a hundred years (it was developed somewhere between the 1910s and 1920s by Dr Edmund Jacobson), involves tensing and relaxing muscle groups progressively and is designed to reduce physical tension at night. That said, as it also involves a bit of concentration I would say that it also works through distracting the mind, albeit to a lesser extent than the cognitive distraction strategies.

The whole process should take about 15–30 minutes and I usually suggest doing this just before going to bed once you have mastered the technique. The key point here is to reflect on the difference in sensation(s) between when your muscles are tensed up and when they are relaxed. Start at the top, with your forehead. Tense up your forehead, as if you were really puzzled or surprised, then count to five. Then slowly, over a count of ten, relax your forehead.

Once your forehead is relaxed, focus for a second or two on the difference between tensing and relaxing and how your forehead feels now. Then move to your eyes. Scrunch them shut, hold for five and then release over a count of ten. Remember to focus on how that felt before moving on to the nose. Again, scrunch your nose up, like you have smelt something bad, and then slowly relax. Then move on to the main facial muscles – the lips, chin, cheeks – and scrunch, relax and review, as before, all of them together (as if you were showing serious disapproval or dismissiveness).

Then move to the shoulders, arms and hands, repeating the same process throughout (count of five once tensed, count of ten to relax and then review on how it felt). You will then go, systematically, through the chest and abdomen, the hips and buttocks and legs and feet.

Remember to do lots of deep breathing throughout. You can match your inhale breath to the tensing and the exhale breath to the relaxing. This is going to take a little practice and so I would always say to try doing it a couple of times in the daytime, until you have got into an automatic routine, before you apply it at night.

Other Strategies

While we are on the topic of relaxation, I often get asked about recommendations for other forms of sleep 'therapy' that revolve around relaxing the mind or body. I have quite mixed feelings about most of them. In my experience, people, especially those in the thick of the acute insomnia phase, tend to start out at the pharmacy or supermarket trying various lotions and potions, advertised to help with sleep, before discussing their sleep with a GP/PCP or considering CBT-I, if they have even heard of it. So, by the time they have got to me they have tried most things, with limited success. Now, I am not going to say that none of those things work, ever, as the likelihood is that some lotions and potions will have some benefit for a small number of people, but I am always left wondering whether it worked through a combination of the placebo effect, a lucky coincidence of taking the remedy or supplement on the odd reasonable night of sleep and levels of natural remission. All I will say is if it works for you, every time, then go for it.

As for other relaxation strategies, from my experience, playing relaxation tapes, especially ones that involve lots of spontaneous noises (rainforest noises or whale song), can be a little counter-productive. While they could be considered a distraction strategy, and as such, they fit with the overall philosophy of cognitive distraction that I talked on page 138, to me it is not going to be distracting enough, as it is quite a passive activity. Additionally, some people who have tried various relaxation tapes have told me that they are constantly waiting to hear what is going to happen next, which is not conducive to sleep. If anything, a repetitive noise would probably work better, if at all.

The final relaxation strategy that I am going to talk about is yoga. Unfortunately, there is not enough reliable data on whether it works for people with insomnia, or not, but I have to say that it is one technique that I am in favour of but am, sadly, rather ignorant about. Anecdotally, people have reported longer sleep, better-quality sleep and feeling refreshed on waking after practising yoga even for only a short amount of time. Specifically, Kundalini yoga has been used with people with insomnia with some promising, albeit preliminary, results. I certainly think that is an avenue if you are interested.

Day 7 Maintaining Success and Relapse Prevention

As always, we will start with the Sleep Diary. But, for today, what I want to focus on is how far we have come in terms of your main insomnia complaint(s). Let's start by comparing your average SL and WASO, from your Pre-course Sleep Diary, with the averages from the last three days, from your On-course Sleep Diary.

I have chosen the last three days as opposed to just last night because of the issue of night-to-night variability in sleep. As I mentioned earlier, even 'normal' sleepers have a bad night and people with insomnia will have the occasional reasonable night. So, I want to look at a combination of the last three nights so that we do not have too much of an under- or over-exaggeration of where we are now at.

What we should be expecting, if everything has gone according to plan, is that both SL and WASO should now be significantly reduced. How much of a reduction (what we call the treatment outcome in research) should we be expecting? Somewhere around a 50% reduction, or more, on each of those symptoms. Next, you may want to compare the other sleep calculations (SE and TST) from the Pre-course Sleep Diary with the last three days. As your SE should now be firmly aligned to your PTIB, that should have increased considerably compared with what it was from your Pre-course Sleep Diary but should not have changed significantly since we introduced stimulus control on Day 2.

What about your Total Sleep Time? The likelihood is that your TST has not changed much at all as, until now, we have focused on reducing your main symptoms (problems getting off to sleep or staying asleep) and increasing the quality of your sleep. Titrating your sleep rescheduling routine, until you get to your Sleep Efficiency goal, will, given time, increase your Total Sleep Time. The other thing to note here is that TST increases even after the course is completed and you have stopped titrating. Whether this is because of the long-term impact of the other aspects of the course on your sleep, in addition to the sleep rescheduling and titration, we're not entirely sure, but we know that your TST does continue to increase, little by little, even after you have completed the course and reached your Sleep Efficiency goal.

Maintaining Your Successes

We discussed yesterday about continuing, after the course is completed, with your sleep rescheduling but what about all the other techniques that we have used over the duration of the course? Should any of these be continued? And if so, for how long? Before we take each strategy and determine its helpfulness going forward, I would say a couple of things. For some of you, a particular strategy may have been helpful outside the issue of sleep and insomnia. If that is the case, then do continue, as none of the techniques you have learnt needs to be put away forever and if it can be applied to another area of your life that you feel needs some attention, if appropriate, that's a bonus. That said, please don't treat your sleep as fragile, thinking that as soon as you stop doing any technique your insomnia will come back. That is rarely, if ever, the case, or at least it is the one issue that I have never come across or had to deal with. As I mentioned earlier, the more you believe your sleep is fragile, and needs wrapping up in cotton wool, the more likely that you will be forever anxious about it and that is never a good recipe for sleeping well.

Okay, so let's start with sleep hygiene. I believe sleep hygiene is good for everyone to practise, irrespective of whether you are a good, normal or poor sleeper, so I would say stay with it.

If you forget or don't have time to exercise on one day or have a meal within 2 hours of bedtime on another, this should not stress you out, but just be mindful that the more sleep hygiene you practise, the more healthy your sleep will be.

As for stimulus control, if you are now sleeping better then you probably will not need 'the 15-minute rule' or my variation of it, as you should be asleep. As for the other parts of stimulus control, for the moment, let's keep the bedroom for sleep and sex alone and no sleeping anywhere else, except bed, until we have reached our Sleep Efficiency goal.

Next, cognitive control. In my experience, this is the one of the main techniques that people have felt has helped them, beyond 'sleep', with people generally reporting that after completing their Cognitive Control Diary, even for a short while, they have felt a little more in control of their overall lives. If it has that benefit for you then please do it as often as you like. Again, as with sleep hygiene, if you forget to do your diary one evening or you just don't find the time, don't get stressed out about it. You can always put it on your to-do list for tomorrow.

Just like the getting out of bed when you know sleep is not happening, from the stimulus control instructions, there should not really be a need to do your cognitive distraction techniques any longer, as you should be asleep at that time.

Finally, what about decatastrophising sleep? Here again, as with cognitive control, people have reported using it outside of the sleep/insomnia context with some good results. Certainly, if you do get overly preoccupied with something, an event, circumstance or issue, and you start to develop catastrophic thinking about the consequences of that situation, you may find this a great way to refocus your mind. Almost like being able to see the wood – the bigger picture – and the trees – each individual worry and concern – for what they actually are.

The final thing on the issue of maintaining your successes is what to do when you have reached the balance between your Sleep Efficiency goal and your feelings of being alert and refreshed when you wake up. What should you do now?

Well, there is certainly no need to keep titrating, as you have reached the optimal point of matching your sleep need to your sleep opportunity. The most important thing at this point, and going forward, is to maintain, as much as possible, a stable sleep/wake schedule around your final Prescribed Time in Bed, which of course includes your final Prescribed Time to Bed and Prescribed Time Out of Bed, the most important of all being your Prescribed Time Out of Bed. As I said on page 111, a stable wake time helps keep the sleep homeostat and sleep/ wake circadian rhythm working in concert.

Again, don't treat your sleep as if it were fragile but also don't start treating it as a commodity that can be traded or abused. That to me is just good sleep health. Maintaining a stable sleep/ wake routine is invaluable armour for good sleep health but I do understand that life sometimes gets in the way. If you slip up and don't go to bed and get out of bed at exactly the same time, again, don't get stressed out. Think about it this way, one night of sleep rescheduling did not 'fix' your insomnia and so the likelihood exists, all things being equal, that one night when you go to bed outside of your new routine is not going to open the gates for insomnia to come flooding straight back in.

So how many nights of 'deviation' from your PTIB can you have? I would say two in a given week, with one main caveat. The reason I have chosen two nights is because of the diagnostic definition of insomnia. There has to be at least three nights, per week, of sleep disruption for it to be classified as insomnia and, as such it makes logical sense, at least to me, to stay underneath that threshold. So, as for the caveat – there are two actually (sorry).

Firstly, deviations should be pre-planned and never used as a compensatory response for a bad night (what to do in those circumstances comes later, on page 161) and, secondly, and lastly, these deviations should be planned with a set time limit in mind (say anywhere between an additional 30 minutes to an hour in bed).

Finally, when you have reached the point that there is no more titration needed there is one other thing I will recommend, something nice for a change. You can now start to incorporate some things back into the bedroom, if you wish, within reason. For example, if you like to read in bed then taking a book to bed is fine again. I would prefer electronics still not to be used in the bedroom, including the television, but re-introducing pleasurable activities that don't involve blue light, work, food and/or exercise should be absolutely fine to do.

Preventing a Future Episode

The next thing we need to talk about is how to prevent the problem from happening again. But first, let's be clear, if you get insomnia again, it is not that same insomnia that you had before coming back and you have not somehow 'relapsed into that same episode'. It is in fact, and as the research tells us, a case that once you have had an episode of insomnia, you are more vulnerable to it happening again in the future. Why does this happen? We are not entirely sure but we know it happens, a lot.

One theory, my own, is that your very first episode of insomnia creates an initial 'wound', for want of a better term, to your sleep system (the sleep homeostat and/or sleep/wake circadian rhythm) and that leaves a scar. As with most scars, there is always going to be extra sensitivity around the affected area, which makes you a little more vulnerable in the future. That is, as I have said a few times throughout the book, not a reason to treat your sleep as fragile forever more. The reason I say that is that it is also my belief that this vulnerability scar pertains to having a sleep disturbance and not to having insomnia per se. As such, I believe that – and, again we have some good evidence to support this statement – by identifying the risks beforehand, and with a little bit of early management, any new sleep disturbance is likely to go as quickly as it came and not be able to develop into acute or chronic insomnia. I believe there are two key processes to consider when thinking about relapse prevention – identifying when you might be at risk and managing the risks in both the short and medium term. Remember I asked you at the very beginning to create your personalised version of Professor Spielman's model (page 59)? Dig that out, as this is where we can use it to both identify and manage the risk of it happening again.

Identifying Risk

As I said on page 3, at some point, most likely within the first two weeks of the sleep disturbance, unless it is managed, we transition from this stress-related sleep loss (sleep disturbance), where the focus is on the stressor, to a point where the sleep loss becomes the stressor (acute insomnia). I call this the sleep-stress switchpoint and it is before this transition (to acute insomnia) that we want to stop it.

Here we are focusing on two different types of risk: proximal risks and distal risks. Together, these look a lot like Professor Spielman's precipitating factors, from his model, but in this instance we are not talking about the sleep disturbance or the insomnia, per se, but rather the stressor itself. In this case, proximal risks are events, circumstances or situations that can trigger a stress response, whereas distal risks are the ways in which our beliefs, behaviours and way of coping can keep the stress going. For example, a break-up can be very stressful but blaming yourself, worrying or becoming obsessed about the break-up is likely to make you feel worse, fuel the stress and make you vulnerable to a sleep disturbance.

Managing Risk

In terms of proximal risks, the truth is you simply can't avoid them and still have some semblance of a life. Again, going back to Professor Spielman's model, the onset of a sleep disturbance is, in most cases, a normal biological reaction to a stressor – either a major life event, a build-up of lots and lots of minor irritations or complications or a constantly stressful set of life circumstances with little respite. So, telling you to avoid any kind of stress in your life is just plain unrealistic. What we can do is identify those trigger points, specific to us, that are likely to result in a period of sleep disturbance. That knowledge alone will give you a sense of control but also give you a benchmark to know when this form of sleep disturbance is 'normal' and when it needs some form of early management.

Going back to your version of Professor Spielman's model, what precipitating factors did you identify as relating to your insomnia? You have them written down and those should serve as the benchmark for what types of precipitating events can cause you to have a stress response that results in a sleep disturbance. Next, think about other stressful events, situations or circumstances that you have encountered in your lifetime that have not resulted in a sleep disturbance. Write a list of them down, next to where you have put your precipitating event(s). Identifying these events serve two purposes: broadly, they tell you that not all stressful events are likely to result in a sleep disturbance but also they give you an indication of the variety of stressors that you have encountered that have not resulted in a stress response.

Of course, we need to take age into account. When we are younger we are all probably a little more resilient to stress, but that is not likely to be the sole reason you did not have a stress response to those other stressors but did have a stress response to the precipitating event that resulted in your insomnia. In essence, working out and writing down what you feel the difference between those events (those that did and those that did not evoke a stress response) provides you with a way to identify proximal risks that are more or less likely to impact on your sleep.

There are, however, some circumstances where a sleep disturbance can be caused by a proximal stressor that has arisen due to a quick change in the homeostatic drive and/or in the sleep/wake circadian rhythm. In these instances, there may be ways to alleviate the problem from the very beginning (within the first few days) or even prevent it from happening at all. For example, there are many medications on the market, both prescribed and over-the-counter, that can either disrupt your sleep or make you feel sleepy during the day. If this happens (you start taking a new medication and you notice within the first few days that your sleep is impaired or your daytime levels of sleepiness increase) it is worth a 'medication management' discussion with your GP/PCP or pharmacist. Questions worth asking include: 'Is this a normal side-effect?', 'How long should I expect this side-effect to last?', 'Are there alternative medications I can take which will not create these side-effects?', 'Is the mix of medications I am on creating the problem?' and 'Is there anything I can do about the timing that I take my medications which might help reduce their impact on my sleep or daytime sleepiness?' These questions can be an invaluable 'first step' in managing the potential for an initial sleep disturbance before it even has a chance to start.

Alleviating the Problem of Jet Lag

The other area where a level of early management can be really helpful is in the case of jet lag, which is a form of sleep disturbance that, believe it or not, can easily turn into a case of acute insomnia. Jet lag is a circadian disruption whereby your biological clock is out of alignment with the timing of the environment you find yourself in. This is due to a rapid change in time zone. As such, your body will want you to sleep at a time that you should be awake and alert. On page 13 I talked about the three exogenous factors that can disrupt the sleep/wake circadian rhythm (light, food and exercise). Here, these things can be used to alleviate the problem of jet lag before it even begins. The key is to align those three things as much as possible to the environment that you will end up in and put those changes into practice a day or two before you travel.

For example, if I am flying from New York to London, let's say on 15 August, there will be a 5-hour time difference. So, I will start eating and exercising, as much as is practical and possible, as if I were on London time from 13 or 14 August.

In terms of light, that is a little more difficult to manage as I do not want you to sacrifice sleep so you can get up earlier than normal (in this example, 5 hours earlier) to get the same amount of light as you would be getting if you were in London. That said, you could certainly control your levels of darkness by wearing blue light-blocking glasses or even sunglasses a few hours before your usual bedtime. Light, I find, is something that you can do more with when you arrive in London. If you arrive in London after sunrise, get out into natural light as soon as possible, try to avoid napping and go to bed at your usual time. If you arrive after sundown then try to avoid natural light, avoid napping and go to bed at your usual time.

Identifying and Managing Distal Risk

However, in most cases managing our responses to the proximal stressor is key in terms of preventing a sleep disturbance from developing into acute insomnia. Where we can have the greatest impact therefore is in identifying and managing distal risk. There has been much research in the area of coping and we know that the style of coping you use, especially to manage stress, can largely determine the extent to which, and the ways in which, the stress can affect you. Research has shown that those people who tend to cope with stress by worrying, getting annoyed or angry (especially with themselves), or ruminating over it tend to have worse outcomes, including sleep disturbance, than those who either distract from it or try problem solving instead. It is important to mention that distraction is not the same thing as denial; it is just ensuring that the stressor does not take over every waking thought. Moreover, those who tend to use substances (for example, alcohol or caffeine) to help manage their stress also tend to have worse outcomes than those who do not.

Here you can apply one of the techniques you learnt on page 133, albeit retrospectively, to identify any distal risk patterns that you may have. You can use constructive worry time, with a slight variation. Next to the precipitant(s) you identified from Professor Spielman's model, write down what you did about it. Again, as before, in this column you can label it as red – nothing at all, yellow – something but later on, green – something immediately. That could have been an action of some sort, a change in the way that you looked at the situation or even ignoring the situation.

We know that the sleep disturbance happened anyway so the distal strategy that you used was not optimal and, at the very least, did not reduce your risk of developing insomnia. So let's reappraise how you coped with that precipitating event now. In retrospect would it have been better to have done: red – nothing at all, yellow – something but later on, green – something immediately? Looking back with an objective mind, you will probably be able to identify what, if any, distal risk patterns you may have and whether they were helpful or not. That is the starting point from which you can apply the principles of constructive worry time in the future. When it occurs, assess the stressor; look at what distal risk patterns you have used, successfully and unsuccessfully in the past, and adopt only strategies that fit with that stressor.

Managing a Sleep Disturbance

On page 3 we talked about sleep disturbance as anywhere between three days to two weeks. Also, we made the distinction between a sleep disturbance and acute insomnia for one main reason – biology. When we talk about stress from a biological perspective we are generally referring to the 'fight-or-flight' response. In most cases this is a normal and natural biological reaction that allows us to manage the stressor at a limited cost to the organism. Whether that management includes more time to deal with the stress, a keener sense of surroundings and threat or increased speed, strength or accuracy, in essence, we are channelling the rest of our existing resources to manage the threat(s) we are facing.

So if a sleep disruption is, as we suspect, a normal biological reaction to stress, how do we manage our sleep during this time? The key here, believe it or not, is to do nothing. As we saw in Part 1, insomnia tends to take hold because of the things we try to do to compensate for it. So, there are the two very simple rules for managing a sleep disruption:

1. Do not compensate for a bad night – keep your wake-up time the same, every day, irrespective of how much sleep you got last night. Remember, you will be increasing pressure on the sleep homeostat while keeping the sleep/wake circadian rhythm regular and in alignment with the homeostat.

2. If you do compensate for a bad night by extending your time in bed (at either end) or by napping in the daytime – pay it back. If you go to bed an hour earlier than normal then push your bedtime back by an hour the following night. However, remember the 5-hour rule. Do not compensate by going under 5 hours of sleep.

Managing Acute Insomnia

As I discussed earlier, after a couple of weeks into a stressor, the biological imperative to reduce sleep should have passed. In essence, the organism (you) will be running on reserve energy and the need to reach biological homeostasis (balance) will become the biological imperative. As such, for most people the sleep disturbance will go away naturally, especially if you do nothing, but some will go on to develop acute insomnia. In this case, managing the insomnia behaviourally – using stimulus control (see Day 2) is the most effective way forward. Here all the same rules for stimulus control apply both in terms of only using the bedroom for sleep and sex, not sleeping elsewhere and leaving the bedroom if you reach the point that you know you are not going to sleep. If you find after a week of doing stimulus control you are still having problems sleeping, then I would add sleep rescheduling (as long as you do not have Paradoxical Insomnia and are good to do this after going through the algorithm). Remember to use your Pre-course Sleep Diary after doing a week of doing stimulus control as the indicators for your new Prescribed Time to Bed and Prescribed Time Out of Bed and never to go below 5 hours' Prescribed Time in Bed.

Conditioning to Good Sleep

As we discussed on page 55, insomnia can be maintained by 'conditioned arousal' to the bed and bedroom environment. So, can we use this information in a positive way? Absolutely, but it is important to do this only when you have a sustained period of normal sleep, say six months. In this instance, repeatedly pairing a stimulus with a positive sleep response (sleep) strengthens the association between the two so that, eventually, with enough pairings, the stimulus will automatically generate the conditioned response.

I will demonstrate with an example from my own life, which has worked pretty well for me: I love the book *The Devil Wears Prada* by Lauren Weisberger. During a period of relatively good sleep – of course, there was the odd night or two of poor sleep mixed in – I would get myself ready for sleep and then start reading the book. Over the first few nights I got quite far into the book but, by the end of the second week I never got to the end, as I would be fast asleep after re-reading where I had left off the previous evening. These days, when I am having an odd poor night of sleep, I will pick up the book and now even opening the book starts to induce sleepiness.

Does the stimulus have to be a book? Not at all, pretty much anything can be conditioned within reason. Some colleagues I have spoken to about this mention using a favourite movie. The things I would tend to avoid are things that can physically or psychologically stimulate you – caffeine, food, exercise, blue light or work, for example. Otherwise you will be pairing something that wakes you up with sleep, which is not the association we are looking for.

Other Helpful Techniques

As always, start with your Sleep Diary calculations; yes, even when you have completed the course. You should, if needed, still be in the titrating phase (unless you have Paradoxical Insomnia) although now you will just need your TIB and TST numbers to work out your Sleep Efficiency in order to continue to do the titrating weekly, as necessary. In this section I am going to focus on a couple of additional techniques, some I have used quite frequently with a great deal of success, although they do not come as standard with a CBT-I package or indeed with the course.

As you have reached this stage of the book, you should have been through the algorithm and been okay to continue. This is important before trying either of the techniques that I am going to share with you. The reason that I am emphasising this again at this stage is because there are individuals with certain conditions who should NOT use either of these techniques as it could make their symptoms worse. So, if you did not meet the conditions for doing the course (i.e. either you do not meet criteria for insomnia or you cannot take part because of a specific illness or condition or medication use) you cannot substitute these techniques for doing the full course and should discuss your sleep with your GP/PCP, consultant or a Behavioural Sleep Medicine specialist.

The two main techniques that I am going to introduce to you are paradoxical intention and a brief version of mindfulness for sleep and insomnia. The reason that I have specifically included paradoxical intention is because in 1999 the American Psychological Association, based on a review of the existing data, recommended its use for people with insomnia. Mindfulness for sleep and insomnia is included as I feel it can be very beneficial and, although only relatively recently applied to people with insomnia, the data supporting its use is impressive.

Neither of the techniques is here to replace parts of the course; they are mainly here to use if you would like to try something different. The one thing I would say is that paradoxical intention and mindfulness for sleep and insomnia should not be tried until after you have completed the course. The reason for this is that, although both of these techniques are complementary to most of the other techniques that we have discussed, the things that we will be asking you to do for paradoxical intention and mindfulness for sleep and insomnia work in a very different way to how the cognitive distraction strategies work. As such, if you tried doing all three things (paradoxical intention, mindfulness for sleep and insomnia and cognitive distraction) together, it will get pretty confusing very, very quickly. Mainly, I use one of these techniques when someone that I am seeing for their insomnia does not get on very well with cognitive distraction. They have had to have tried each of the different cognitive distraction strategies first but, if they cannot get to grips with any of them, that is when we change tack. Okay, on to each strategy.

Paradoxical Intention

Paradoxical intention, to me, provides a fascinating insight into the quirkiness of the human mind. This technique, in the context of insomnia, was created by Professor Colin Espie. If you remember, he originated the term Sleep Effort (see page 55) and that is exactly what paradoxical intention is designed to combat.

Let's start with a small experiment. I want you NOT to think about a purple elephant. What are you thinking of? Most likely you are thinking about a purple elephant. So the behaviour that I have asked you not to do, you automatically have done and the likelihood is that you could not help it. This is what we mean by paradoxical.

Let's now apply that to sleep. Think about the most boring event that you have ever had to go to in an evening. Perhaps a dinner party with the dullest people you have ever met or a bad movie at the cinema or the theatre where you were just wishing the performance to end. Have you ever found yourself, during that boring evening, saying to yourself in your head, 'For goodness sake don't fall asleep ... don't fall asleep ... don't fall asleep'? The likelihood here is that you are going to nod off, albeit briefly, when you tell yourself to stay awake ... again paradoxical. So, if the behaviour we are looking to elicit is to fall asleep, what should you do paradoxically? Stay awake.

The most important thing here is not to actively TRY to stay awake; that is effort, which will lead to physical tension, but to just stay awake for a little bit longer. So, get into bed, as normal, turn the lights out and get everything ready for sleep. However, I want you to keep your eyes open for this. Now, let go of any thoughts about getting off to sleep; instead ask yourself to stay awake for just a little bit longer. You will start to notice, pretty soon, that, just as in the case of the boring evening, your eyes will start to feel heavy and you may find yourself unable to stop yawning. It will be tempting to shut your eyes at this point but don't; just ask yourself to hang on to wakefulness for just a little bit longer. That is it. The great thing is this technique can be applied if you wake in the night as well as during the period of getting off to sleep. So, how long should you do this technique for? I would say if you get to the point that you realise sleep is not coming, as you would do under stimulus control instructions (when you realise that sleep is not coming get out of the bed and bedroom, if appropriate, and only return after 30 or 45 minutes), then stop.

Mindfulness for Sleep and Insomnia

Here we will look at a very different approach to managing unwanted thoughts, worries and ruminations at night. But first, a couple of individuals must be acknowledged, Professor Jon Kabat-Zinn and Dr Jason Ong. Professor Kabat-Zinn pioneered Mindfulness-Based Stress Reduction (MBSR) and I would thoroughly recommend his book *Full Catastrophe Living* if you would like to learn more about mindfulness in general.

Dr Ong, on the other hand, has done pretty much all of the work examining mindfulness techniques in people with insomnia. The way Dr Ong incorporates mindfulness into CBT-I is interesting and underscores why I feel it should not be attempted until after you have completed the whole course. He uses mindfulness alongside psychoeducation about sleep (in essence, Part 1 of this book), sleep hygiene, stimulus control and sleep rescheduling (sleep restriction). The traditional cognitive components are generally not included (i.e. cognitive control, cognitive distraction or decatastrophising sleep) in a mindfulness-based version of CBT-I. The reason being is that, as you will see in a minute, mindfulness for sleep and insomnia is attempting to address the negative thoughts, worries and concerns we have about our insomnia and its daytime consequences in a very different way to the 'traditional' cognitive therapies.

There are a couple of things to discuss from the outset with mindfulness for sleep and insomnia. The first is that it takes time to learn and lots of practice. Most of the studies that have been done to look at how well it works for people with insomnia (alongside the behavioural techniques from CBT-I) involve at least six, if not eight, sessions, in addition to a full- or half-day workshop which includes meditation exercises. I was recently asked by someone with insomnia why it would take so long. This person went on to ask why I could not just recommend one of the 'mindfulness colouring-in books' that she had seen instead. I have nothing against those books personally, but I am not really sure they are fully embracing all the principles of mindfulness. Instead, I am more inclined to say that these, in the main, from my experience of flicking through a few, are centred on mental relaxation and/or cognitive distraction. As such, I did not recommend a mindfulness colouring-in book, as mindfulness is not, in my understanding of it, attempting to change your levels of tension per se.

The second thing to note about using mindfulness for sleep and insomnia is that you should do all your practice during the daytime and only apply it at night when you feel confident. This level of practice usually involves 30–45 minutes per day, 5 days a week for 6–8 weeks and practice should not be done within 2 hours of bedtime. What the research does show, however, is there is quite a strong relationship between how much you practise mindfulness for insomnia and how well it works.

So, as I mentioned, mindfulness for sleep and insomnia takes an altogether different approach to traditional cognitive therapy for insomnia. Instead of working against sleep-related thoughts, feelings, worries and concerns, as we do with cognitive distraction, we are going to work with these thoughts, feelings, worries and concerns instead. This should not, however, be seen as a passive approach but rather an adaptive response which puts our sleep and insomnia into perspective. Here, I am going to outline seven main ways from which you can re-examine your relationship with your sleep, your insomnia and any sleep-related daytime sleepiness or dysfunction you experience. Whilst this is NOT the full mindfulness technique as has been applied by Dr Ong in the context of insomnia, these are the principles that I feel are important when considering how we can change our relationship with our insomnia and reduce sleep-related worry.

Non-judging – don't judge being awake at night as an automatically negative occurrence. It is a neutral concept and should be acknowledged as such. Similarly, don't judge being sleepy in the day as an automatic negative occurrence, it just is that. Feeling sleepy in the day. There have been times when we have needed to sleep outside 'normal' hours. For example, when we have not been very well. Under those circumstances we did not see the sleep we got then as necessarily negative, it just was.

Beginner's mind – treat each night as a single entity. Have no expectations about your sleep tonight based upon what has happened during the day or indeed the sleep you got last night or the night before. On page 3 I ranted on as to why I don't like the term 'insomniac'. I felt it gave your insomnia an identity. This is similar in the sense that the more history you attach to your insomnia the more that the whole (the insomnia) has become greater than the sum of its parts (your sleep). Thank you Aristotle!

Non-striving – reduce your effort to sleep at night and your need to hide or combat any feelings you have of daytime sleepiness. They both exist and should be acknowledged for what they are, nothing more, nothing less. Expending a great deal of effort trying to manage our sleep and the consequences of your insomnia gives it an identity. This way of dealing with effort is very akin to paradoxical intention. The other issue is, when we strive for sleep, we also tend to ignore the bigger picture. It is very common for people with insomnia to cancel social engagements or activities, which are pleasurable, in an attempt to get more sleep and/or manage daytime sleepiness. Cancelling those engagements however is neglecting a different aspect of your overall health and wellbeing.

Acceptance – accepting your present state. For example, saying, 'Yes, I did not sleep very well last night and, yes, I do feel tired or sleepy today.' These are legitimate thoughts, which you can observe and accept without the need to act upon them.

Letting go – this is not about avoiding a thought or trying to clear your mind. Allow your thoughts to come and go as they please. Make a conscious decision to accept any sleep-related thought and feeling for what it is; a thought or feeling, and don't try to change, problem-solve or suppress the thought or feeling. It is a much better thing to acknowledge the thought as a thought without attaching any evaluation to it. Try acknowledging the thought by telling yourself that you are thinking, as opposed to focusing on what the thought might mean.

Trust – knowing that your mind and body are not out there, or in this case, in there, deliberately trying to destroy you or are so dysfunctional that they are doing you damage through mismanagement or neglect. Trust that your body and mind can and will regulate both your sleep and daytime needs if you let them. Think about it this way: new parents suffer a significant amount of sleep loss for quite long periods of time but under most 'normal circumstances' they do not fall apart. Similarly, even after a prolonged period of sleep deprivation, it takes a relatively short time for the body to recover and for sleep to go back to 'normal'. This is evidence that your body and mind have the capacity to self-regulate and correct for sleep loss and you need to ultimately trust that they will do their job.

Patience – understanding that the quality and quantity of your sleep will not improve overnight and this new approach will take time and practice.

This approach was not easy for me to grasp at first, as it was so alien to my training and my rather rigid established ways of thinking and working. One of the ways by which I have found mindfulness for sleep and insomnia easier to understand is by looking at the parallels with the concept of stress. Stress tends to have very negative connotations. If I say the word 'stress' to you, it is usually interpreted as something bad has happened or is about to happen. However, at its most basic physiologic level, cortisol (the 'stress hormone') is actually neutral. Cortisol is produced by the adrenal cortex and, while it is true that more is produced when we are under challenging circumstances, we need a certain level of cortisol to live and function. In fact, cortisol serves several vital functions to keep the body in balance. It helps us metabolise fat, carbohydrate and protein and helps regulate our blood sugar and insulin levels. Even when it is deregulated, as in the case of challenge, the increase in cortisol is there, in part, to ensure an appropriate response by the immune system. As such, cortisol itself is a largely neutral or adaptive response but it is how much emphasis we place on it that can make it 'stressful'.

PART 3

Case Studies

In Part 3 I am going to introduce you to a few case studies that either I, or one of the trainees whom I have provided supervision for, have encountered over the years. The reason for Part 3 is that, unlike the case study in Part 1 (Lydia, on page 52), most of the cases that we see are complex and yours may well be too. Therefore Part 3 is designed to provide, through each example, some helpful guidance if you have what appears to be insomnia alongside another illness or condition. Naturally, everyone's experiences will be different but it may be beneficial to see how the process works from our perspective.

I have changed the names and any identifying details (for example, occupation, family status, living arrangements) of each patient to protect the innocent (that would be me). What you will notice is that the background section in each case study is very similar. I, and my trainees, use a rather formulaic approach, even before we get into what the problem(s) are with an individual's sleep and what predisposing, precipitating and perpetuating factors may exist. The reason we do that is that the information that we get at that point really does give us clues as to what may be either causing the problem or making it worse and, of course, if there are other issues we need to look at first. I have outlined this approach in the table below, so you can follow what I am doing. The reason that I am sharing this with you is that if you do see a Behavioural Sleep Medicine specialist they are likely to go through a similar set of questions with you, so you can prepare.

Personal factors	Age
	Sex
	Relationship status
Occupation	Working hours (or history)
	Working pattern
Household	Who lives in the household
	Who or what regularly sleeps in the bedroom
Health status	Body mass index
	Physical health history
	Psychological health history
	Current physical health
	Current psychological health
	Medication use
	Substance use (including over-the-counter medications)
	Sleep history
	Family sleep and health history
Lifestyle	Exercise
	Diet
	Alcohol use
	Caffeine use
	Smoking
	Morningness/Eveningness preference
	Hobbies and interests
Stress levels	Work stress
	Home stress
	Other stress
	Coping style
Bedroom factors	Bedroom environment
	Bedroom routine
General sleep pattern	Work-day and non-work day patterns
	Patterns while on vacation
	Typical number of hours sleep

Case Study 1: Rob

Background

Rob is a 34-year-old painter for a multinational construction company that builds luxury homes. He is in full-time employment. He does not do shift work but regularly works over 40 hours a week, sometimes doing additional private jobs for people in addition to his 'usual' workload. He has a long-term significant other (Jo), one child, aged six (Mallory) and two dogs (Sam and Salty). The dogs do not sleep in the bedroom.

His body mass index (BMI) is 27 and he describes himself as a 'little bigger than the average bear'. He has no history of serious physical or psychological illness, or head injury, and does not have any chronic illnesses presently and is on no prescription medication for a long-term condition. He also has had no sleep problems in the past. Although, to his knowledge, neither of his parents have had nor currently have a sleep problem, his father has hypertension for which he is medicated. Rob does not do any formal exercise although he does say that his work does keep him 'fit enough' and Mallory keeps him pretty busy at the weekend. He does not smoke but drinks a pint, or two, of lager on most nights but will drink more with his work colleagues on a Friday night (approximately five–six pints of lager). His caffeine intake is a bit high. He does not drink coffee or tea but will have four, 'or more', diet cola drinks a day, with his last caffeinated drink to go with his supper. He takes no other substances. His diet is 'reasonable', if not a bit heavy, and he puts this down to Jo being a 'great northern cook' although they will get a takeaway at least once a week. Rob and Jo will eat supper usually around 7 or 7.30pm.

He describes himself as a 'bit quiet', but reasonably happy with work and life. He states that his general stress levels are 'fine' and he reports 'just getting on with stuff' when stress does happen.

The bedroom is generally cool but he can tell when it is day-light through the curtains and there is some noticeable traffic noise, from the street outside, more so in the late evenings when he goes to bed. Rob and Jo go to bed around the same time and he feels that they are both moderate evening-type people. His general sleep pattern is quite variable, especially on days off, and he will go to bed anywhere between 10pm and midnight. He does not read or watch TV in the bedroom and the only electronic gadget in the bedroom is his phone, as he needs his alarm to get up. The phone is readily accessible next to the bed and he checks it if and when he wakes up in the night. At the moment (as sometimes Rob has to travel different distances to get to the site he is working at) Rob has to be up at 5.30 to get ready on work days and on non-work days Rob will get up somewhere between 8 and 10am, depending on Mallory. On average, Rob is getting about 5½–6 hours sleep a night.

Presenting Complaint

Rob's main issue is that he feels that his sleep is unrefresh-ing and he gets really exhausted during the day because he wakes up a lot in the night. He states that it takes him 'no time at all' to get off to sleep but he is awake during the night, several nights each week, for over an hour. These awakenings are numerous (at least four or five) but he does get back off to sleep within about 15–20 minutes. He states that he does not ruminate during these awakenings but will lie there quietly not wanting to disturb Jo. He says there is no specific pattern to his sleep problem, although it is more noticeable at weekends, and the awakenings don't happen at the same time every night.

Rob says the current problem started about 18 months ago when he was off from work for a couple of weeks due to an accident he had. He said that he had tripped on a scaffold and damaged his ankle, which left him in quite a bit of pain. He says the ankle in now fine and there was no permanent damage or need for surgery and he is in no pain now. He says that he feels that his sleep problem is impacting on his work and he has been late for work more than a few times in the last year, which is not like him. It was Jo who suggested that Rob see someone about his sleep as she has noticed that his snoring has increased in terms of frequency and volume and on some nights it is so bad that she will sleep downstairs on the sofa. He has tried nasal strips for his snoring and a throat spray but neither made any difference according to Jo. Rob has not been to see his GP/PCP about his sleep or his snoring. When asked about his thoughts about the bedroom, he says he has none in particular, good or bad. It is just a place to sleep. He says he is not overly preoccupied with his sleep throughout the day although he is worried about driving home from work in the afternoon because of his tiredness. In terms of how he manages his sleep problem day to day, Rob will mainly try to get an early night whenever possible or try to 'catch up' on his days off. He says he does not need to nap and has not unintentionally fallen asleep. Finally, Rob believes that he needs at least 7 hours 'uninterrupted' sleep to be refreshed.

Is It Insomnia, Something Else or a Bit of Both?

This is a good question; Rob appears to meet all the six criteria for Insomnia Disorder (middle insomnia). He has a pattern of precipitating events (accident) and perpetuating factors (increased time in bed) but there are some things in what he has said that need further investigating before we can say definitively what the problem(s) are. The snoring is the main issue holding up the diagnosis of insomnia. We need to work out whether the snoring is part of a bigger issue. The other thing is that Rob mentions that his sleep problem is worse at weekends and that may be due, in part, to the increased alcohol which will make his snoring worse. What makes this all the more intriguing to me is that Rob did not report any conditioned arousal to the bedroom or bedroom routine and no sleep preoccupation or catastrophic thinking. That is unusual in insomnia but not unheard of.

Initial Impressions

The first thing we need to do is get Rob a referral to check for any sleep-related breathing disorders. While he is waiting for his appointment we can start recording his sleep, with a Sleep Diary, and look at sleep hygiene. Now, as I always say, sleep hygiene is not going to fix the problem, as it is very unlikely that poor sleep hygiene caused the problem in the first place. That said, when Rob does get checked we want his sleep hygiene to be good so that we can get a clearer understanding of what precisely his sleep problem(s) might be. Specifically, Rob can make some changes to his bedroom environment (light and noisy), put the phone somewhere where he cannot easily get to it to check the time at night and reduce his alcohol and caffeine intake, especially close to bedtime. Now, I would not do CBT-I, or indeed suggest Rob starts this course, until his results were back from the tests, any actions needed are taken and he gets an all clear from his GP/PCP or specialist. The other thing I would not do at this time is ask Rob to try to keep to a regular sleep/wake schedule, even though I would in a lot of other cases, as if he does have a sleep-related breathing disorder he may need that extra time in bed, until he is treated, just to keep him awake and alert in the day.

Outcome

A specialist saw Rob about his snoring and he did an overnight test at home (not full polysomnography). His Apnea/Hypopnea Index came back at seven, which suggests mild Obstructive Sleep Apnea (OSA) – see page 65. Rob was referred to a dentist who specialises in Mandibular Repositioning Appliances (MRAs). A MRA is something like a gum-shield, which is worn in the mouth at night. It helps by keeping the airway open, which not only helps with the OSA but reduces the snoring as well. MRAs are generally used for mild to moderate apnea or if the individual has more severe apnea but cannot tolerate a Continuous Positive Airway Pressure (CPAP) device (more about that below).

Additionally, some lifestyle changes, including regular exercise, making some changes to his diet and reducing his alcohol intake were also advised by the specialist. At his follow-up appointment, a month after Rob was given the MRA he was asked how he slept on nights where he used his MRA. Firstly, Rob noticed how this question was framed and stated that he uses his MRA every night without fail. It took him a couple of nights to get used to it but it now is part of his routine. In terms of his sleep, Jo has noticed the snoring has reduced quite a lot and she no longer has to go to the sofa and Rob states that his daytime sleepiness levels have dropped significantly. That said, Rob is still experiencing frequent night-time awakenings, which is still causing him some distress.

As Rob is compliant with his MRA and the specialist and GP/PCP feel that he is ready for us to treat his insomnia, we can go ahead, which we do. As is appropriate, we (including the GP/PCP) discuss all the options with Rob, pharmacological and non-pharmacological, and he chooses a full CBT-I treatment approach. The one thing that we had to be extra mindful of when we were doing CBT-I in this case is monitoring for any significant increases in his daytime sleepiness levels. Rob is now sleeping much better with only the occasional wake-up during the night (once or twice a month), usually to use the bathroom. Case closed.

Continuous Positive Airway Pressure

Continuous Positive Airway Pressure is generally used for cases of more severe OSA or when there is OSA and additional evidence of excessive daytime sleepiness. A specialist, usually in Respiratory Medicine or ENT (Otorhinolaryngology), will prescribe CPAP after testing for sleep-related breathing disorders. CPAP comes in many shapes and sizes although generally it involves a mask, which fits over the nose or nose and mouth. The mask is connected to a motor by a tube and the motor produces air pressure that keeps the airway open, preventing partial or full collapse of the airway. Many people feel the benefit of CPAP almost immediately with reduced sleep disruption and snoring and increased energy during the day.

Case Study 2: Kathy

Background

Kathy is a 58-year-old former hotel receptionist. She retired three years ago on the grounds of chronic neuropathic pain. In the past she did shift work, but says that it never bothered her. She now spends her time in helping out her daughter by looking after the grandchildren during the day and she meets up with friends whenever she can. She is a widow and has two children (Michelle who is 35 years old and Michael who is 32 years old). Kathy lives with her new significant other (Roger) and they have no pets and neither child lives at home. Kathy has a BMI of 20. Her health status, outside of the chronic pain, is good and she has no other physical or psychological illnesses or conditions. She had a relatively early menopause (started when she was 47) and was prescribed hormone replacement therapy (HRT) but she came off HRT three years later. Kathy has no history of head injury or any other psychological or physical illnesses. She is prescribed Gabapentin for her chronic pain in three daily doses, which she takes in the morning, afternoon and just before bed. She reports that the Gabapentin has helped with the pain overall but she does still have pain twinges, particularly in the early evenings. Although she was only diagnosed with chronic pain three years ago she has been in pain for the last five years. She takes no other substances.

Kathy says she has always been prone to sleep disturbances, particularly when she is under stress, but nothing in the past has been like this in terms of severity or length. With regards to family history, Kathy noted that her mother was always a poor sleeper. Additionally, her mother, who passed away three years ago, had type 2 diabetes and cancer and her father has been diagnosed with asbestosis. He lives nearby and Kathy 'pops in' every day to deliver shopping or 'to make sure that he eats something healthy'. In terms of lifestyle, Kathy drinks only at weekends and that will be one or two small glasses of wine, and she goes swimming twice a week but is not fanatical about it. She also enjoys her weekly yoga class although describes herself as 'less than perfect' at it. She does not smoke but drinks at least four cups of coffee a day, with her last coffee at lunchtime. She says that her diet is good and she rarely eats takeaways although she reports to be a 'sucker for a good dessert'. Her dinnertime is usually around 7.30pm. Kathy says that her stress levels are 'manageable' and the yoga really helps. She went on a meditation course a couple of years ago and says that this is how she manages any stress and when the pain gets really bad. Kathy has read up on sleep hygiene and her bedroom is cool, dark, quiet and comfortable. She has nothing distracting or arousing in the bedroom and only uses the bedroom for sleep and sex. She does use an alarm clock, as she likes to keep to a regular wake time, which is 7.45am, even at weekends. Her night-time routine is usually going to bed around 10pm unless there is something 'good on the television, which is rare'. On average, Kathy is reporting getting about 6 hours sleep a night.

Presenting Complaint

Kathy reports her main problem is being awake for long stretches in the night. On average she wakes up two or three times during the night but these awakenings can last an hour to an hour and a half each time. These awakenings occur 'five nights out of seven' and have been going on for about eleven years. Kathy says that her sleep problem started around the same time her menopause started and she would have hot flashes during the night, wake up 'drenched' and have to change the sheets. Since the sleep problem started Kathy says there have been very few periods of remission, if at all. Kathy states that these awakenings are random and there is no difference in pattern at weekends or when she is on vacation. When asked what she would do when she was awake, she replied that she tried to meditate but usually found this difficult and would end up dwelling on 'odds and ends'. She would stay in bed during these times as she felt it was better to be resting than 'up and about' at that hour.

When asked to talk about her sleep and her bedroom she described the 'dread' of going to bed and how she would get anxious even before she started getting ready for bed. It is difficult for Kathy to definitely say whether her sleep problem is interfering with her life, because of the pain that she experiences, but she certainly says she is distressed by it. She has no other concerns about her sleep, although Roger snores sometimes and she has to 'tell him nicely' to move on to his side. Roger has nothing to add in terms of Kathy's sleep and has not noticed anything odd or unusual in terms of behaviour or restlessness. Over the years Kathy has tried numerous alternative remedies from the supermarket but nothing has helped. She has discussed her sleep with her GP/PCP and was offered sleep medication, which she tried at the beginning. She says that it provided some relief, but soon wore off and she did not bother to get a repeat prescription. Kathy believes that her sleep problem and pain are linked and this combination is going to make her seriously ill in the long term, like it did to her mother. She does get preoccupied with her sleep during the day but finds the meditation and yoga help a lot with that. She has tried napping during the day but just cannot do it. Finally, Kathy feels that she probably needs 8 hours of sleep to feel refreshed.

Is It Insomnia, Something Else or a Bit of Both?

This looks like a case of both. Kathy already has a diagnosis of chronic pain and meets all the criteria for Insomnia Disorder (middle insomnia). What we know is that pain causes sleep problems and sleep problems decrease our capacity to tolerate pain. That said, the sleep problem started before the pain and so the likelihood is that the pain is adding to an already existing sleep problem, possibly through increased cortical arousal. She has a pattern of predisposing, precipitating and perpetuating factors. Specifically she is spending quite a lot of time in bed, nearly 10 hours a night, and a lot of that time she is awake. She also demonstrates conditioned arousal and lots of sleep-related preoccupation that she is trying to manage.

Initial Impressions

As Kathy meets all the criteria for insomnia and the pain, albeit an issue, is not adequately explaining the insomnia we can move forward. Now, Kathy is already seeing a pain specialist and is on Gabapentin. This is where we need to get everyone on the same page before we go any further into the issue of how we manage the insomnia. We need to make sure that there is going to be no conflicting advice given between the GP/PCP, the pain specialist and us. It is quite common, especially in conditions whereby there is chronic pain (such as in the case of fibromyalgia) or when there is significant fatigue (such as in the case of cancer and especially during the treatment of cancer), for advice to be given about resting and daytime napping which may conflict with the traditional non-pharmacological treatment of insomnia (such as traditional CBT-I and this course). As Kathy's sleep hygiene is excellent we don't really need to do anything with that other than, perhaps, remind her that it is good and to keep it up. I would also recommend her completing a Sleep Diary.

Outcome

A series of discussions were had between all four parties (Kathy, us, the GP/PCP and the pain specialist). The pain specialist was intending to start a programme of Cognitive Behaviour Therapy for Pain Management with Kathy and the GP/PCP felt that pain management was more of a priority than managing Kathy's sleep problem. As part of our discussions we also explored alternatives to both the Gabapentin and the timing of the last dose, but eventually it was agreed that this should remain as is. Further, the GP/PCP was happy to prescribe a different kind of sleep medication, one that Kathy had not had before over the period that she was going to do the CBT for pain. Kathy did not want to go down the pharmacological route, even as a short-term measure. We, on the other hand, wanted to start looking at her sleep and doing CBT-I.

Now, this is where there is a little bit of an issue as one of my rules is that an individual should not be undergoing two 'lots' of Cognitive Behaviour Therapy, albeit focused rather differently, at the same time. That is not to say that I don't like working in multidisciplinary teams, I just think that it can get too confusing for a patient if they are undergoing two very similar treatments at the same time. To me, that is like being given two similar medications, one for anxiety and the other for depression, where there is one medication that works for both conditions.

In this instance we reached what I believe was a nice compromise. We trained the pain specialist in how to do CBT-I and introduced them to the research of Dr Carla Jungquist and Dr Nicole Tang. Both Carla and Nicole have developed variants of CBT-I that incorporate pain management techniques specifically for people with chronic pain, with great success. The pain specialist delivered a full course of CBT-I alongside their CBT for Pain Management and we consulted with them throughout. Kathy's sleep has improved immensely and although she does still wake once or twice a week, she gets back off to sleep with ease. She also has no fear of the bedroom or of a new sleep disturbance happening in the future. Case closed.

Case Study 3: William

Background

William is a 22-year-old student, studying full time for a degree in mathematics. He is doing well 'mostly' at university and it looks like he will graduate with honours. He also works part time in a local bar four nights a week to supplement his student loan. He has a good social life and has lots of friends both at home and at university. He lives in shared accommodation, near campus, and has a bedroom of his own. There are five other people who live in his building and he says that he gets on with them all 'okay enough'. He has a significant other (Ibrahim) and they spend two to three nights together a week, usually at William's place. William has no pets. His BMI is 18. His physical health is good and he is on no prescription medication for any long-term conditions. He has suffered from both anxiety and depression in the past but is, at the moment, not taking any medication for either condition. He has no history of major physical illness or head injury. Presently, he says his mood is 'spiky' and he gets the feeling that something bad is about to happen quite frequently. This has been going on for the last month but he has not sought help from his GP/PCP, as he wants to 'ride it out'. He has tried cannabis in the past but presently does not use any substances.

He describes his sleep history as 'okay' although he has never been a good sleeper. He does not know about his family's sleep history as they don't tend to talk about 'health stuff' but his older sister (Jean) was diagnosed with chronic fatigue syndrome a year ago. William's exercise regimen consists of playing badminton once a week and 'lots' of walking across campus. He states that his diet is poor and he will have takeaways several times a week as he considers it 'cheaper in the long run'. His last mealtime is very variable, depending on his work and university schedule, and can be anywhere between 9 to 11pm. He does not smoke but does drink alcohol, mainly on the nights when he finishes work at the bar. His intake of alcohol is variable but will usually consist of a couple of pints of lager or cider on those nights. He does drink caffeine and will usually have two cups of coffee a day but only in the mornings. He says his stress levels 'should not be as big as they are' but feels that he lacks the necessary coping skills to manage the demands of both work and university. As he predominantly lives in one room, his bedroom environment is also his living and studying environment. He says he has no control over the thermostat and it is either freezing cold or boiling hot in his room. The room can also get noisy, from his housemates as they all work and study on different schedules and he presumes that he makes just as much noise for them. The room is dark, when needed, and he cannot tell if it is morning when his curtains are closed. Naturally, there are plenty of electronics in the room with his laptop, tablet, phone and games consoles all being within 'easy reach'. William says he 'needs' his alarm clock to get him to where he needs to be every day otherwise he would be late.

He says that he is an evening person and will generally go to bed when he feels tired. This can be anywhere between midnight and 2am. On some days he has to be up and out by 8.45am but on days that he does not, he will sleep in till about 11.30am or noon. On average, William is reporting about 7 hours of sleep a night.

Presenting Complaint

William is having problems getting off to sleep. On average it is taking him an hour to 2 hours to get off to sleep, despite feeling tired. He says that he is exhausted all the time but just cannot sleep when he tries. His sleep problem started about six months ago and, although he cannot put his finger on a particular event that triggered the problem, around that period he was 'stressed all the time'. He feels that his sleep problem is impacting on his ability to concentrate at university and is concerned that his grades will suffer if his problem continues. When asked what his sleep pattern is like on days where he does not have university or work, or during the summer break, he said that he would generally sleep lots more, sometimes not 'surfacing' until the middle of the afternoon but would still feel sluggish. William has no other sleep complaints and says that no one from where he currently lives or his family has suggested anything odd about his sleep habits except for his 'vampire-like behaviour'. He has not tried anything in the past to manage his sleep problem as he was hoping it would just go away, eventually.

When asked what he would do during those hours that he was trying to sleep, he said that he would initially just lie awake and start to worry about university and his performance. He would also try harder to fall asleep but eventually, when this failed, he would get his laptop out and start doing assignments. He reports being preoccupied with his sleep and this makes him even more anxious during the day. When asked what he felt about his room, William said that he 'hates the way he lives' and sleep is 'just a painful experience'. Finally, William feels that he needs somewhere between 8 and 9 hours of sleep a night to feel refreshed.

Is It Insomnia, Something Else or a Bit of Both?

It looks like there may be potentially three, or more, things going on here. Although William has all the symptoms for a diagnosis of Insomnia Disorder (initial insomnia) there are several complicating factors, which prevent me from that immediate conclusion.

His age, alongside the late nights and, when he can, late mornings, suggests a potential Circadian Rhythm Disorder (delayed), which is more common than we realise in adolescents. We know that adolescents need more sleep than adults but something else happens when puberty hits. The production of melatonin starts to delay and we tend to become more and more evening oriented. Because of this delay in melatonin production the cues to sleep (such as yawning) are also delayed, if present at all at this stage, and so we prefer late nights and late starts in the morning. That is why teenagers can be hard to wake up in the morning. It is not laziness but a biological change that does not quite fit with a lot of young people's school or university schedules. This process can last right into the middle of our twenties. However, if we take all that into account alongside William's work/university schedule, he may also have some sleep deprivation, as he is not getting his ideal sleep need for this time in his life. This may explain why he still feels sluggish when he does sleep a lot (during the summer holidays) as he is still paying off the sleep debt that he has built up during the semester.

There is also William's mood to take into consideration and that needs investigating further as sleep onset problems can be a sign of issues with anxiety. That said, there are all the hallmarks of Insomnia Disorder, including plenty of sleep effort and sleep preoccupation/catastrophic thinking, and the fact that the sleep problem came before the anxiety leads me to think that the anxiety is not causing the sleep problem but probably making it worse.

Initial Impressions

The first thing we need to do is look at William's sleep/wake circadian rhythm before we can tackle the insomnia, if the insomnia actually exists. We also need him to talk to his GP/PCP about his anxiety as, even if he does have a Circadian Rhythm Disorder and/or insomnia, CBT-I or this course would be harder to tolerate with anxiety on top. That is not to say that, and if his GP/PCP agrees, we cannot start with the course until after the anxiety is managed; we would just need to take some extra precautions.

The issue of sleep hygiene is, in this case, a little complex. As William lives essentially in one room we need some creative thinking around ensuring his bedroom is cool, dark, quiet, comfortable and free from easily accessible electronics. What I advise in this situation is similar to what I said on page 127 about people who, for whatever reason, could not leave the bedroom at night when they were doing sleep rescheduling and stimulus control. Here, designate two separate spaces, a day space and a night space. Electronics should stay in the day space. If he could get a screen or sheet which would separate the two that would be even better. As for cool and quiet, keeping the windows open and earplugs may be the best ways forward. We also, at this point, would talk to William about how alcohol and eating late affects his sleep.

Outcome

We gave William an actigraph and a Sleep Diary to monitor his sleep for two weeks. During that time and where possible, he was to sleep *ad libitum* as much as possible so we could compare his sleep/wake circadian profile between 'work' and 'non-work' days. In the meantime, William agreed to talk about his anxiety symptoms with his GP/PCP. It worked out that William did have a significantly delayed sleep/wake circadian rhythm, more so than we would expect at this time in his life, and as such had a Circadian Rhythm Disorder. The CRD was treated, in conjunction with a specialist in chronotherapy, using light therapy, which took a little bit of time. Although William's GP/PCP was happy for him to start the course to manage his insomnia before his appointment with a specialist in anxiety came through (William did not want to medicate for his anxiety), by the time the light therapy was concluded he no longer met criteria for insomnia and so the full course was not necessary.

William was now sleeping to a regular schedule and the sluggishness that he experienced was all but gone. He was, however, still anxious about his sleep. What we did do was talk to William about sleep effort, identifying risk, using the Spielman model as we did with you (page 59), and prevention in terms of sleep disturbances. Case closed.

Case Study 4: Sally-Ann

Background

Sally-Ann is a 59-year-old retired business accountant. Although she no longer works full time, she still does 'the odd consultancy contract' for the firm that she had worked for previously. This, she states, takes up one day a week of her time, 'at most'. She has never done shift work. She occupies herself during the day by doing 'the books' for a local charity and she is very keen on golf, playing at least three times a week. She has an active social life and is 'always out' in the evenings, or at least until recently. Sally-Ann is single and lives alone. She has no pets, 'even though she adores animals', as she is allergic. Her BMI is 17. She was diagnosed with having an over-active thyroid (hyperthyroidism) when she was 40 and had her thyroid removed within a year and now takes Levothyroxine every day at breakfast time. More recently she was diagnosed with iron deficiency anaemia and is taking iron supplements twice daily. Apart from that, Sally-Ann reports no other physical illnesses and a good physical health history. She came through the menopause 'relatively unscathed a few years ago'. She is on no substances.

She has had no problems with her sleep in the past and considered herself a 'great sleeper' until the problem started. She does not believe that either parent suffered from any sleep problems and both parents lived into their eighties. Shortly after her mother died of a heart attack (unusually, she did not have coronary heart disease), her father developed dementia and he moved in with Sally-Ann. She cared for him, in addition to working full time, for approximately five years. He passed away four years ago, which is around the time that her sleep problem(s) first started. She saw the GP/PCP for depression at the time of her father's death and was prescribed a Selective Serotonin Reuptake Inhibitor (SSRI). She came off the SSRI gradually over the next year but says that her mood has been 'variable' over the last six months.

Sally-Ann gets lots of exercise, mainly at the gym, sometimes into the late evening, says she has a 'good diet' and does not smoke. Her last meal is at 8pm. She does drink alcohol and will have a large glass, or two, of wine on most evenings and 'perhaps one more' if she is out with friends. She will also have the odd glass of whisky on nights that she 'just knows' she is going to have trouble sleeping. She also drinks coffee but only in the morning, then she switches to tea. Her last tea intake is 3pm. Sally-Ann says her stress levels are 'not particularly high, except on days after a poor night's sleep' and describes herself as an 'undeniable, uncontrollable perfectionist' and says she can be quite critical, but only about herself. Her bedroom is cool, dark and quiet. She has a television in her bedroom, which she watches when she is awake in the night. She also takes her mobile phone and tablet into the bedroom and will also use them during the night. Sally-Ann likes to keep to a sleep/wake routine and will 'almost always' be in bed by 11pm and up at 7am, irrespective of what she has on the next day. She will read for about 30–40 minutes in bed and then will try to sleep. She says she gets, on average, 4½ hours of sleep a night.

Presenting Complaint

Sally-Ann says she has no difficulties getting off to sleep but has difficulties with both waking in the night and waking too early in the morning. On average she says that she wakes up twice a night, always in the very early hours – 2am(ish) and around 3.30 – and is awake during the night for a total of 2½ hours and then will wake up around 5.30 in the morning and not be able to get back off to sleep. She says this pattern happens frequently, about four times a week, but there is no specific pattern of exact times that she wakes up.

She says the problem started four years ago but it appeared to get better after about a year. After almost a year of sleeping better the sleep problem started again. The present episode has been on going for two years. The trigger, for the first episode, as we saw earlier, was the death of her father but she cannot recall anything specific that has made her sleep problem 'come back with a vengeance'. When prompted on this, she did say that around the time the sleep disturbance came back she was having the house remodelled as she had made a lot of adjustments to the house when her father came to live with her and it was 'a bit chaotic'. She feels the sleep problem is impacting on her mood and she is cancelling social engagements more and more as she feels that she would not be good company as she is so tired. She does not feel that she has any other sleep problems and has never been told that she is excessively restless during sleep or that she snores. That said, more recently she has noticed that her bed sheets are 'all over the place' in the morning. She has tried several relaxing tapes but they did not appear to help and just made her more frustrated. She has not discussed her sleep with her GP/PCP. When asked what she thought of the bedroom she said that it is still a 'lovely room' but she just 'does not like being there like she used to'. Sally-Ann says that she does sleep a bit better when she is on vacation but this is 'short lived'. She also reports that thoughts of sleep do 'get in the way' and she is worried that this is now permanent and she will have to learn to live with this level of poor sleep due to her age. She feels that she probably needs 7 hours of sleep to function the next day.

Is It Insomnia, Something Else or a Bit of Both?

Sally-Ann does, on the face of it, look like a clear-cut case of Insomnia Disorder (mixed middle and late insomnia). She meets all the six criteria and does outline a pattern on predisposing (perfectionistic personality, previous episode of insomnia), precipitating (the remodelling of the house) and perpetuating (sleep preoccupation and conditioned arousal) events and circumstances. There are, however, a couple of things I think we need to follow up on at the same time.

Firstly, the average amount of sleep that Sally-Ann is reporting is getting very close to the limits I set for detecting Paradoxical Insomnia. Secondly, I am always curious about messy beds in the morning. While a dishevelled bed could be a sign of a restless night of sleep, it could also be indicating Periodic Limb Movement Disorder (PLMD). As we have some anaemia in the mix, late-evening exercise and alcohol being used to sleep as well, all of which can make PLMD worse, I would not rule it out. The SSRI is also an interesting issue for me, as we know that some SSRIs can increase the symptoms of PLMD and when Sally-Ann came off the SSRI she did have a period of remission. The current mood also needs some thought and attention. Waking early in the morning can be a sign of depression and Sally-Ann said her mood has been 'variable' for the last six months. Although the change in mood has come after the sleep problem, it still needs some form of investigation to see if it will impact on any other treatment strategies.

Initial Impressions

The first thing we need to do is find out the extent to which Sally-Ann's sleep problem(s) could be due to all the things that affect PLMD, and of course, whether she has PLMD. Also, we need to know whether Sally-Ann has Paradoxical Insomnia, or not. We also need to ask her to get her iron deficiency anaemia checked with her GP/PCP to see if she needs to increase the iron supplements and also talk about the recent change in her mood. There is nothing stopping us from starting Sally-Ann on the Pre-course Sleep Diary and sleep hygiene, as they will be helpful to the GP/PCP and us. Specifically for sleep hygiene, we need to address the use of alcohol to sleep, the electronic use in the bedroom and the exercising close to bedtime as the main issues. As this is a complex issue, with lots of potential influencing factors, we are going to have to take a systematic step-wise approach, tackling one thing and then the next and so forth.

Outcome

The first thing we did was asked Sally-Ann to make an appointment with her GP/PCP to discuss her mood and her iron deficiency anaemia but not to discuss her sleep specifically at this juncture. While that was being organised, we asked Sally-Ann to do a quick experiment. Here we asked her to stop drinking alcohol and exercising in the evenings, just for a week, and to keep a Pre-course Sleep Diary during that time. We also asked to keep a track of her 'messy bed' during that week and start sleep hygiene. At the end of that week Sally-Ann reported that her sleep was already better, with fewer prolonged awakenings and no messy bed, but she was still waking significantly earlier in the morning than she needed to.

She then saw the GP/PCP and was tested for iron deficiency and her mood was discussed but nothing was agreed between them in terms of treatment. The following week we asked Sally-Ann if she would be okay if she continued her experiment for another week (in other words, no alcohol and no late-evening exercise) while we monitored her sleep with an actigraph. Here we were looking at the potential for Paradoxical Insomnia. During that week the results came back from the GP/PCP and both her iron levels and binding levels were fine. The results from the week of actigraphy came back and there was no sign of significant Paradoxical Insomnia. As Sally-Ann still met all the criteria for Insomnia Disorder and there was no evidence of PLMD or Paradoxical Insomnia, the next step was for Sally-Ann to discuss treating her insomnia with her GP/PCP. We spoke with the GP/PCP, on their request and with Sally-Ann's agreement, and the GP/PCP gave Sally-Ann the go-ahead for us to treat her insomnia. Sally-Ann chose a brief face-to-face version of CBT-I (in other words, this course with my physical presence). Her sleep and her mood have improved greatly and now she sleeps through the night and wakes up with her alarm at 7am. Case closed.

Follow-on Note

The one thing I would note here, and that Sally-Ann's case highlights, is the impact that treating insomnia can have on mood. Several studies, including one of my own, have shown that one of the 'by-products' (and I call it a by-product because we are not entirely sure why it happens) of CBT-I, and courses like this one, is that it impacts on our mood. Both the symptoms of anxiety and depression appear to reduce significantly following a CBT-I treatment. This is a very recent and, at least to me, exciting scientific finding and although we are only just starting to understand it, it certainly makes me happy (a huge shout out to Dr Colleen Carney and Professor Rachel Manber for doing this exceptional work).

Talking Sleep With Your GP/PCP

On a different tack, let's look at talking about sleep with your GP/PCP. Sadly, across the globe, education about sleep medicine is very limited, especially for what I call 'front-line' medical professionals (those who work in Primary Care). Although there are a couple of medical specialities (such as psychiatry and neurology) that do have some sleep medicine education embedded into their core training, the likelihood is that your GP/PCP will largely be working from prior experiences with patients as opposed to an in-depth knowledge of sleep medicine per se. I am not going on a witch-hunt against GP/PCPs, as I believe they have enough on their plate but this is a simple truth. The first thing to remember is that your GP/PCP is also likely to be aware that their knowledge-base is limited with regard to sleep medicine in general, and behavioural sleep medicine in particular, as several studies in the UK, Australia and the USA have already demonstrated.

Here is where I feel you have a real opportunity to work together. This is also one of the reasons why I have suggested that if you have a sleep problem, and by using the algorithm on page 33, you determine that it is either not insomnia, or is insomnia but complicated by another situation, condition or illness that needs management first, you should complete the Pre-course Sleep Diary and start doing sleep hygiene before you see your GP/PCP. Taking your Sleep Diary with you to your appointment alongside the knowledge that you already have good sleep hygiene will save both of you time and energy from the beginning. That way you can move forward with assessing and managing your sleep. Hell, take this book as well if you think it will help.

One of the things I would like you to think about, in advance of the meeting with your GP/PCP, is to not get overly focused on any 'other' illness, condition, medication or substance. That is not to say that those issues should be excluded from the conversation altogether, as they are very important and, in part, why you are there, but there may well be a temptation for everyone to focus exclusively on another illness or condition, keeping everyone in his or her comfort zone. Another reason I say this is because for a very long time insomnia was seen as a secondary symptom to another illness and, although that has now changed, at least in terms of the diagnostic algorithms that I talked about when we looked at the definition of insomnia, it may be the case that your GP/PCP still believes that. Remember, when we looked at the diagnosis of insomnia, the term 'adequately explains the insomnia' comes into play here. If the insomnia started around the same time as the 'other' condition or circumstance and is not being successfully managed then the other 'illness' may well be explaining the insomnia and that will need further investigating. If it is not the case then the insomnia should be examined, assessed and treated in its own right from the outset but following an assessment of the impact of this course on that illness or condition, and vice versa.

How to Locate a Good Behavioural Sleep Medicine Specialist

A lot of what I am going to say in this very final part of the book depends upon where you live, both in terms of number of specialists available and ensuring they are appropriately qualified and/or experienced.

I will be upfront about this from the beginning: finding a Behavioural Sleep Medicine specialist (BSM) is going to be a bit of a challenge, either for you or your GP/PCP. The reason for this, sadly, is that BSM is a largely undefined profession. While the United States of America, Australia and Europe have made significant progress in terms of standardising BSM training and identifying potential career pathways for BSM specialists over the last few years, there is still a great deal of work to be done.

So the Internet will be a really invaluable tool at this point as finding a good BSM is going to involve some investigative work. While most BSM practitioners will (at least, they should be and you should check to make sure) be credentialled, and regulated, by a professional body, under a particular speciality (for example, medicine, psychology, counselling, nursing, midwifery or social work), they are unlikely to be credentialled solely as a BSM.

If someone suggests that they are only credentialled in BSM, to me that is a red flag. I am not suggesting you run screaming from their office but I would probably like to know more about that person's training and experience before I part with any time or, if applicable, money.

How Good Is Their Training?

So, how do I determine whether their training was any good? Again, this is where some investigative work needs to be done. There are some amazing CBT-I training courses out there (I teach on a few of them) and some not so amazing ones (which I do not teach on). The key here is to find out who ran the course and do some background research on that person as well as on the content of the training course. Oh, and don't take what is said on the advertising website as gospel, go deeper.

The first thing I look for is whether the trainer has published any papers, specifically on the topic of CBT-I, in scientific journals. You will find that most, if not all, the 'grandfathers and grandmothers' of CBT-I have, and many papers at that. If and when you ascertain that your BSM has attended a recognised and respected training course, then I would ask to see some recommendations or, even better, meet a former patient. This may not be possible because of confidentiality issues but it never hurts to ask. I have many people who are more than happy to discuss their treatment with someone looking to undertake either full six–eight-week CBT-I or shortened versions, like this one, with me.

The reason that I am so passionate about this is for two reasons. Primarily I want people to get better from CBT-I, including courses like this one. CBT-I works, in the main, but if it is done badly the likelihood is that the individual receiving treatment is not going to say it was a bad therapist – as, in many cases, how would they know? – but is more likely to say it was a bad therapy.

The other, albeit related, reason is that a bad therapist makes all us Behavioural Sleep Medicine specialists look bad. I remember being called by a very upset GP/PCP a year or so ago, who was bemoaning all BSMs. They had a patient who had seen a 'BSM therapist' (not me, I hasten to add) privately for CBT-I. The patient was in a wheelchair but the 'therapist' still enforced full 'traditional' stimulus control in which the patient was instructed to get out of bed and go to another room after 15 minutes of being awake. Sheer stupidity if you ask me, but you get my point.

The good news is that a few years ago the European Sleep Research Society (ESRS) created an exam, which, if you pass, qualifies you to use the title Somnologist: Expert in Behavioural Sleep Medicine. While this qualification is not solely focused on CBT-I and, as such, you may find a Somnologist who does not deal with insomnia, the likelihood is that, if they don't practise CBT-I, they will be able to recommend someone who can help you. Even if you determine that your sleep problem is not insomnia, they will be able to help or recommend someone who specialises in your sleep problem. The ESRS provides a list of qualified Somnologists on its website and that, to my mind, is the best starting point if you live in Europe.

Along a similar vein, in the USA there is the Society for Behavioural Sleep Medicine (SBSM), which also holds a register of qualified specialists. For other parts of the world, most should have a Sleep Society and a Dental Sleep Society and those should be your starting point.

INDEX

Page references in *italics* indicate tables and graphs.